The Beginning is Sh*t

An Unapologetic Weight Loss Memoir

SUZANNE CULBERG

The Beginning is Sh*t: An Unapologetic Weight Loss Memoir
by Suzanne Culberg

ISBN (paperback) 978-0-6452749-0-5
ISBN (ebook) 978-0-6452749-1-2

Editing by Laura Gates-Lupton
Branding by Emma Veiga-Malta
Book design by DTPerfect.com

Contact the author at **www.suzanneculberg.com**

To my husband Jeremy, who never wavers in his unconditional support.

And

For you if you ever doubt that you're enough. May these words help you uncover the magic within.

Table of Contents

Prologue

This is the story I have always wanted to read.

Every time I went on a weight loss endeavour I would devour before and after stories like I had previously devoured chocolate. I could not get enough of them.

But as much as I loved them, I also hated them. Because they were picture perfect, like a Disney movie, they showed how terrible the main character's life was 'before' and then how perfect it was 'after'.

Then the story would end, and we never found out what happened after the after? Did the main character stay slim and healthy forevermore? If so, what was her secret? Because that was never the case for me.

My weight went up and down more often than a roller coaster. Surely I couldn't be the only one? Where were the stories like mine?

So now I get to share it with you.

For anyone reading this I just want to say, this is my story, from my perspective, with my lens and focus.

It's never my intention to paint anyone as the 'bad guy'.

I realise that we all do the best we can with the resources we have available at the time.

Revisiting this story with the viewpoint I have now I can totally see a different perspective.

But in any story who is right anyway? Doesn't the saying go, there's my version, your version, and then what really happened?

I say this as a reminder that whatever happens to us in our lives, we can choose to stay stuck in that story, or we can choose to take the lesson from it and move on. I hope my story helps you to transform your own x

Note: Aside from myself, my husband Jeremy and my children Xanthe and Casimir, all names have been changed.

Prequel

The dressmaker is trying her best to yank the dress down over my head, but it's stuck at the armpits, and it won't budge. I suck in my stomach and try to wriggle into it like I have seen my Mum do in the past, but still no luck.

"That's it." Mum says. "You're going on a diet." — I am 4.

Chapter One

EARLY YEARS
1989

"I'm sick," I say to Mrs Spelling.

"You're not sick, go sit on the mat," she snaps.

"I am sick. I am on medi," I reply in a small voice.

"It's medication!" she proclaims. "You're at school now. We don't use baby language here. Get to the mat NOW!" she ends with a shout.

I hate it when she shouts. I run over to the mat crying.

I don't understand the rules of school.

I have never been in anything like this before. When I want something, I have to raise my hand. I learn this part fast. But what I don't understand is why I have to wait for 'recess' or 'lunch' to go to the toilet. At home I can go to the toilet whenever I need.

"I need to go to the toilet," I say.

"You need to hold until recess," Mrs Spelling says.

"But I am busting," I whine.

"You're at school now. You go at recess or lunch. Now go join the circle," she says.

I drag myself over to my spot in the circle. We are singing and dancing to the farmer in the dell. I really need to go to the toilet. I try to hold on, but when we start dancing I can't hold any longer and I wet myself. There is a circle-shaped wet patch on the carpet.

Everyone laughs at me.

I am not sure what to do, I look down at the ground feeling my cheeks get hotter.

"Wait there," Mrs Spelling snaps, as she marches over to the cupboard to get out the spare undies she keeps for when someone has an accident.

From that day on Mum starts packing me spare undies in my school bag. She doesn't understand what the issue is; I don't wet myself at home.

I learn that if I say I am sick, I get to stay home a lot. So I start pretending to be sick. Eventually Mum cottons on to this and makes me go to school regardless.

One day I really am sick, and no amount of pleading with Mum will let me stay home. I get to school and I am still saying I'm sick but she ignores me. It's a sports day and we are supposed to be running around the tennis court.

"Go and run," says Mrs Spelling.

"I can't, I'm sick, I want to go home," I say.

"Go and run NOW!" she insists, raising her voice.

I vomit all over her shoes.

Every now and then we get to have movie day at school. Mrs Spelling will wheel in a tv set on a stand and pop in a video for us to watch. These are usually my favourite days at school, it's such a treat to watch a movie. One day we watch a movie about bigfoot.

From that day on I am scared to go outside. I am forever worried that bigfoot will get me. I have a lot of nightmares about this. It reaches the point where my parents or sisters have to check it's 'safe' before I go outside, and I refuse to ever go outside by myself.

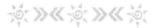

We are getting fitted for our dresses for my oldest sister Cara's wedding. I am to be the flower girl. My other sisters Claudia and Chloe get to be bridesmaids.

Cara is buzzing around the room, telling everyone what to do, as usual. At only four years old, my dress is a pink and white number with puffy sleeves and flowers sewn on it.

I don't like it.

It's different than everyone else's. Their dresses are all pink. I want my dress to be all pink too. I don't like that mine is different. I don't like that I am a flower girl and they get to be bridesmaids, I want to be a bridesmaid too!

My mum and sisters are flipping through bridal magazines and discussing hair options, so I'm left to be measured up with the seamstress.

"Look, Mummy, I'm a big girl," I say, sucking in my tummy like I see my Mum and sisters do whenever they try on clothes.

They don't look up from their conversation, and the dressmaker takes all of my measurements. I'm so proud of myself for holding in my stomach like a grown up. I'll have to remember to tell them again later.

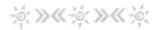

A few weeks later when the dresses are ready, we're nervously sitting in my sister's lounge room, waiting to be blown away by how amazing we all look. Cara is inspecting my two sisters' bridesmaids' dresses up close, preening and picking over every inch.

Then it's my turn.

The dressmaker is trying her best to yank the dress down over my head, but it's stuck at the armpits, and it won't budge. I suck in my stomach and try to wriggle into it like I have seen my Mum do in the past, but still no luck.

"That's it." Mum says. "You're going on a diet."

I don't know what this means, but I hope we can go soon. I'm really bored, and I want to watch cartoons.

On the way home from the dressmaker we call into the supermarket and buy 'diet' foods, skim milk, mandarins, low-fat yogurt and vegetables.

When we get home, Mum begins to clean out the kitchen, throwing out all of the 'bad' food. I watch as my favourite muesli bars go into the bin, followed by the ice cream and cookies.

"Go play outside," Mum says, as I perch backwards on a kitchen chair watching her going through all the items in the kitchen.

"I'm scared of bigfoot, can you check it's safe?" I ask.

"I don't have time. I am getting things organised for our diet," she replies. So I sit and watch in fascination as she goes through the entire contents of the pantry and fridge.

The diet starts on Monday. For breakfast I am allowed one piece of toast. In my lunch box is packed a mandarin for recess and a vegemite sandwich for lunch.

I am not allowed anything between lunch and dinner.

For dinner we eat meat and three vegetables, usually potato, carrot and corn. For dessert I can have diet yogurt.

We all last on this diet till about Thursday, when Dad brings home honeycomb chocolate and liquorice, and Mum cracks out the tins of condensed milk and dairy milk chocolate.

We gorge ourselves on all the forbidden food! I love it! Friday and Saturday become my favourite days of the week as we eat ALL the stuff that is forbidden during the week.

Sundays suck because it's the day all the goodness comes to an end and we must go through the cupboards once more and throw out all the 'bad' food ready to start our diet again on Monday.

This dieting cycle continues for as long as I can remember living at home.

Different variations but the same result.

Chapter Two

PRIMARY SCHOOL
1992

It's Friday afternoon. "Your assignment is to create a poster displaying your full name, height, weight and your favourite hobbies. Make a start over the weekend and we will measure your height and weight in class next week to finish it off," says Mrs King. She gives us a piece of A3 paper to roll up and take home.

As I walk to my dad's work after school, I dream up all the ways I can make this poster. I think about the glitter and textas I have at home. What can I put down as my hobbies? As an eight year old, I've been reading for a couple of years and love it, so drawing a book is a given. I also love photography; perhaps I can take some photos to include.

I explain the project to Dad and ask if we can take some photos to use. That night we take some photos of me in the sunset and pictures of the view from our house. He prints them out for me the next morning at work.

Saturday afternoon I spend a wonderful time creating the poster with Dad. He encourages me to map everything out in pencil first, then we glue down the photos and erase the pencil to write in texta. I leave blank spaces to enter my weight and height.

On Monday morning I proudly enter the classroom carrying my poster. It is sensational! Quite a few of the other kids have done nothing and are hurriedly scribbling on their posters.

A boy at my desk looks down at my poster and snidely remarks "Your photos are stupid. Who do you think you are, a model?"

It feels like a punch in the gut. Moments ago I had been so proud of my poster, and now I feel a sense of dread. I try to hunch forward and cover my poster as much as I can. Another boy pipes up with "and what is with all that glitter? What are you, four?"

I slump even farther forward and try desperately to cover my poster.

Can I ask the teacher for another?

"Ok, class, it's time to line up and have your height and weight measured to complete your assignment. Line up here, and one by one we will measure your results, and you can take them back to your poster."

I line up, feeling a growing sense of dread. I know I'm big. I don't want everyone to know how big. As the line creeps forward I want to run. I really don't want to do this. Having heard the reactions to my photos and glitter, I can't even imagine the reactions to my weight. I don't understand why we have to do this.

I want to go home.

Eventually I make the front of the line. My height is measured first and I am 122cm, so on the shorter side, but not the shortest. My weight is to be next.

I hesitate before stepping on the scales.

"Why do I have to do this?" I ask Mrs King.

"It's part of the project," she replies.

I stand there looking down at the scales with dread.

"Come along, Suzanne, you're holding up the class," says Mrs King.

I exhale fully first, hoping that by having empty lungs I can remove a few grams, and I step gingerly on the scales.

"32 kilograms!" exclaims Mrs King, her voice raising as she says it. "Are you sure? Dear, step back off and on again, just in case the scales need to reset". I do as she asks, and yes my weight remains the same.

I leave the line with my head down and dawdle slowly over to my desk.

In pencil, as faint as I possibly can I write down my weight and height. Dejectedly I hand my poster to Mrs King at the end of the lesson.

During recess she hangs the posters up on the wall.

The class comes back in after recess to see the results. My poster stands out a mile, the colours, the glitter...I really did put a lot of effort into creating it. Fortunately you can't read the numbers from a distance.

People crowd around the posters and one girl pipes up. "I knew you were fat, Suzanne, but I didn't realise you were the fattest in the class! You're even heavier than Justin!"

Everyone turns to me and laughs. Mrs King tries to change the subject by announcing it's time for Maths. We split up into our maths groups and as we move around the different activities it starts. "Fatty tube sticks" someone whispers.

"Godzilla," says someone else.

I keep my head down, and I focus on my work.

At lunch time, my weight is the talk of the school. The news travels fast, and a boy from grade 6 comes over to me and asks, "How many rolls are in a bakery?" I look back at him confused. He and his friends snigger and saunter off. I don't know what this means.

As if the taunts about my weight aren't enough, there are also plenty of taunts about my middle name. My middle name is Gay, and that starts off a tirade of teasing.

Our teacher tries to calm that down, letting us know that her sister's name is Gaye. But the kids say it doesn't count because it's spelt differently. Her name is Gaye, but mine is Gay, and so that must mean I am Gay. I don't even really know what Gay means either. I don't understand what all the fuss is about.

I can't wait for the day to end. I keep looking at the clock in the classroom and willing the numbers to move faster. As soon as the bell rings after school, I race to my dad's work as fast as I can.

I cry as I run, and I burst into his workplace, tears streaming. My dad is confused. He asks if I have hurt myself and looks me up and down for injury.

I blurt it all out, the glitter on my poster makes it look like a 4 year old did it, the photos make me look like I think I am a model, I am the fattest person in my class and I look like Godzilla, and my name is Gay, so I must be Gay.

"What does Gay mean, Dad?"

My dad explains to me that the other kids must be jealous of me. I had put a lot of effort into my poster, and it made them feel bad. I don't think he gets it. I don't want to go back to school. So much so that I flat out refuse to go. For the rest of the week I stay home.

I start my very first diet of my own, above and beyond my family's haphazard dieting. I also heard that exercise helps you lose weight, so I decide to take up running.

The next day I go for my first run. The ground is very uneven; we live on a property, and I long for the footpaths that the suburban kids have.

I push on, this running thing is going to be my salvation.

It's not long until I get really out of breath. My lungs burn and I can't breathe. I stop running and cough violently.

It hurts to breathe.

I can feel this searing pain in my chest. I go and ask Dad about it. "You're unfit," he says. "Push through the pain and it will get better."

I try this, but it keeps getting worse, and I just can't breathe. I decide walking is better instead. So I commit to walking our driveway every day.

I also watch a television show where a girl throws up and loses weight.

I try throwing up. I put my fingers down my throat and nothing happens. I gag a bit, but I can't make myself sick.

I feel like an utter failure. I can't even make myself vomit.

So back to dieting it is. I swear that I am going to make it this time. I am never going to eat chocolate or lollies ever again. I am going to stick to my diet every day of the week and not just Monday through Thursday.

I am feeling super proud of myself for sticking to my diet. So much so that when Mum says I have to go back to school on Monday I don't mind so much. I am losing weight. I will show those kids.

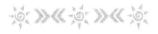

Primary school continues in much the same fashion. Many diets, many kilograms lost and regained.

No matter how hard I try I can never quite stick with it.

I long to be like the other kids who don't have to worry about what they eat.

I am bullied for my weight repeatedly. Sometimes I tell my parents. Most of the time I don't. I dream about the day where this will all be behind me.

Chapter Three

HIGH SCHOOL
1996 - Grade 7

I am in two minds about starting high school.

I am excited to learn more, explore new subjects and maybe make some new friends. But I am nervous that I am going to be the fattest.

I have always been the fattest in my class all through primary school. Will high school be the same? Hopefully with larger class numbers there will be other big people.

I long to make friends with another fat kid. I hope I can find someone else who 'gets it'.

Everywhere I go, the first thing I do is look around and see if I am the biggest person there. Most of the time I am.

There are 3 grade 7 classes. There are 3 fat girls, one in each class. I am disappointed. I wish they had put us all together. So once again I am the fattest in my class.

Asides from physical education (PE) class, I really enjoy all my high school subjects. As part of PE there are 3 all-school sports carnivals — athletics, cross country and swimming.

I dread anything related to exercise.

At the swimming carnival we all must enter the free-style race. I am such a slow swimmer that when I finally finish the race, I notice the winners have already climbed out of the pool.

In the cross country, I am so dead last that the volunteers are packing away the witches hats and markers before I have finished the course.

But worst of all is the athletics carnival. We MUST enter the 100 metre sprint.

The sprint track is directly in front of the stands where the entire school is sitting. I walk up to the track with trepidation.

When the starting blast goes off, I try as hard as I can. I run, I pump my arms, my lungs are burning, but I am way too slow.

I can hear the laughter and the taunts from the stands. "Look at fatty tube sticks run, look at her thighs rub together".

I want to die.

I arrive back to my seat following the race, red faced, coughing and trying desperately to find my bag, when a teacher appears next to me.

"I've just entered you in the hurdles event, grab a drink and get ready," she says.

"No." I flatly refuse.

"Suzannnnnnnne," she says slowly, dragging my name out. "We get one point per race we enter, so chop chop."

"I can't hurdle." I say in a high pitched voice. "I will fall on my face."

"Where's your school spirit? Atta girl, up and at them."

By this stage I'm trying my best to hold back tears. I'm also still recovering my breath from the sprint race, so I am kind of hiccuping and wishing the ground would just swallow me up.

She points at the track.

I refuse to move.

The race starts, and another fat girl is in it. My heart goes out to her. I want to run over and give her a hug.

I don't believe it! She refuses to run!

She stomps her way down the course, kicks over the first hurdle, steps over it, continues to march, kicks over the next hurdle.

I am amazed. Who is this girl? How can she be so defiant? I want to be her. I admire her confidence.

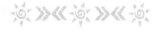

I am bullied in high school.

I can handle the day-to-day stuff. I am used to it.

But in high school I have to catch the school bus. I never had to take the bus in primary school, as I could just walk to my dad's work.

I hate catching the bus.

My bus goes to another school first, so by the time it gets to my school, it's already three-quarters full. I very rarely get a seat. I have to stand in the aisle.

There are a few bullies on the bus, but none is worse than Lorraine.

Lorraine and I went to primary school together. She didn't really bother me in primary school, but in high school she is super mean.

"Are you hungry, Suzanne?" she asks with a gleam in her eye.

"No Lorraine."

"Here," she says, reaching into her bag. "Have some cake."

"I'm good, thanks."

"Are you on another diiiieeeeet?" she asks in a sing-song voice dragging out the word.

Then she grabs my arm and smears the cake all over my blazer.

Mum is going to be angry again because my blazer has to be dry cleaned.

Dry cleaning is really expensive, and we can't afford to keep getting it done.

The blazer is a significant symbol in our house, because I am the only one in the family who attends a private school and gets to wear one.

I must treat the blazer like gold, lest someone see it dirty and my sisters start raging again that I get to go to a private school when they did not.

I learn to take my blazer off before the bus trip and stuff it in my bag.

When my uniform gets dirty, I wash it out by hand in the evening so it's clean for the next day.

Over time, I stop responding to the cake so Lorraine starts to throw fruit at me instead.

I don't mind the soft food like mandarins, but the hard things like apples really hurt.

I won't let them see me cry, though. I save that till I get off the bus, and I run and hide in the public toilets and cry and cry.

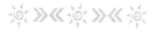

It's not long before my school uniform barely fits me.

I freeze in winter because I can't wear my Rugby jumper as it's too tight. So I have to just wear my polo shirt, even though it's chilly and my fingers turn purple from the cold.

In summer I'm forced to wear my scratchy woollen school jumper because my dress is so tight that the buttons gape too much to be seen without a cover.

The strain at the middle is so much that I worry a button will pop off.

I often fantasise about taking my jumper off on the bus and a button popping off and hitting Lorraine in the eye.

She always manages to get a seat, and I always have to stand.

Mum says she can't afford a new uniform, so at the end of the year I go on another diet.

I once again try purging, but no matter how much I try sticking my fingers down my throat, I can't make myself vomit.

I research ways of making myself puke, and I read that really salty water can do it.

I dump a tablespoon of salt in a small amount of water and try to drink it. All I manage to do is make myself gag.

I try to starve myself, but I always end up way too hungry and then eat whatever I can get my hands on.

Instead I make myself cut out all sweets and go for long walks every day.

Over the summer holidays between ending grade 7 and starting grade 8 I manage to drop 11kg going from 75kg to 64kg.

I am relieved my uniform fits once again!

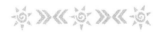

1999 – Grade 10

I weigh myself. 87 kilograms. I am the heaviest I have ever been.

We are standing outside the science labs waiting for class to start. A bunch of the popular girls are standing in a huddle, whispering and giggling. They are nudging each other and looking over at me. I get a bad feeling in the pit of my stomach.

"Hey, Suzanne?" says Nicole.

"Yes?" I reply with dread.

"How many razors does it take to shave your legs?" she asks.

I try to formulate an answer, but I am confused.

"We were just talking," she continues, "and have decided that because your calves are SOOOOOO fat that surely you must blunt a razor before you even finish one leg."

The group of girls begin to laugh.

Angela pipes up with "I reckon you blunt a razor on each stroke." She begins to mime running a razor up her leg and discarding it at the top, and then grabbing another one.

I am finding it difficult to breathe. The rash of despair has creeped up my neck, and I can feel my face is hot.

But also I feel my blood start to boil. I can handle being teased, but this is just stupid. A razor each stroke? I am not ten foot tall, for crying out loud.

"How could I blunt a razor each stroke?" I ask. "My calves may be big, but I am no taller than average. Isn't it the number of strokes that would blunt it, not the length of my leg?"

The rest of the girls begin to laugh, someone sniggers, "Angela just got schooled."

Angela's eyes squint deeply and she glares at me. "Shut up lard ass," she retorts and stomps off.

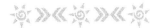

One day in PE class we go on an excursion to Oceana, the local gym.

It's not far down the road from my school and we try a bunch of different group fitness classes. I really enjoy it.

I ask my parents if I can join the gym and walk there after school. They agree.

I am equal parts excited about going to the gym and relieved about no longer having to catch the school bus. I still dread the bus every day, so this is a total win-win.

Although I love exercising at the gym, I still struggle. My lungs burn, and it makes any type of exercise difficult. I complain to my dad about it. He just tells me to push through the pain; it only happens because I am so unfit.

I persist with the exercise. But I am not having great results. I am still complaining bitterly about the pain. So one day Mum decides to take me to the doctor. I am diagnosed with exercise induced asthma. I am prescribed an inhaler and shown how to use it.

It's with great excitement that I attend the gym the

next day with my inhaler. I try out a new class, spin, and I LOVE it! My lungs don't burn, and I can really give it my all in the class.

I push myself so hard that as soon as the class is over I leap off my bike, steady myself on legs that feel like jelly, and run to the bathroom to vomit.

I never thought I'd be excited about vomiting.

Although I know I have pushed too hard, at least I don't feel like my lungs are going to explode.

Over the following weeks I learn the line between pushing myself hard, but not hard enough that I am physically sick.

I begin exploring ALL the group fitness classes. I especially love water aerobics, pump, spin, body attack and circuit.

I love the environment at the gym. It's so supportive. No matter your size, whether you're the biggest or the smallest, and no matter your age, whether you are the youngest or the oldest, you are supported and encouraged to do your best.

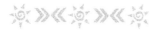

The end of the year approaches, and I am the smallest I have ever been. I have reached 66 kilograms.

I choose a black dress with silver roses for my year ten formal. It is beautiful.

Although everyone tells me how great I look, I still feel fat.

I compare myself to my friends, and I still feel like the 'big' one. I desperately want to lose more weight.

If I can just get to 60 kilograms then I will be happy.

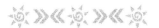

Chapter Four

COLLEGE

In Tasmania, year 11 and 12 are referred to as college and often take place at a separate school.

2000

I am excited and nervous about starting college. I am in the best physical shape I have ever been in, and I am looking forward to meeting new people who never knew the 'really fat' me.

Yet I still feel fat, and I compare myself to my peers constantly.

On the day we go to buy my uniform I am embarrassed that I still need a size 16 skirt.

Most of my friends wear a size 14 and some even a 12.

I feel like such a failure, I have been working so hard, and I am still fat.

My resolve is beginning to teeter, and the food is so tempting.

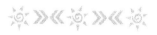

I'm in Life Science class with Mr Rose. Today he is talking about fat cell formation; this has piqued my interest.

With my desperation to keep losing weight high, and my motivation to keep avoiding junk food low, I am on the precipice of throwing in the towel.

Mr Rose explains, "Fat cells are formed before puberty, and once the number of cells are formed there is no destroying them. The fat can leave the cell, but the cell itself won't degrade. So there is a point where a person reaches a weight set point and can't get any smaller."

I feel instantly deflated, what is the point of continuing with this journey when I physically can't get any smaller? I am already working so hard at school, and at the gym, and trying to eat right. I feel like I don't have any more to give. Plus I am not going to get any smaller anyway because my number of fat cells has already been set by younger me who ate too much? This isn't fair!

After school I skip the gym and I go to the bakery. I buy a custard scroll, and I eat the entire thing as fast as I can. After that I go to the supermarket and buy a family block of chocolate. I eat that too. Might as well eat it all, I am destined to be fat anyway. What's the point?

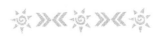

My mum's business is going bankrupt.

The stress is palpable.

We don't have the money for a gym membership anymore so I have to let that go.

The day the shop finally closes Mum lets me take a day off from school, but gives me strict instructions not to answer the phone.

It rings constantly as all the debt collectors start calling us at home.

I am not allowed to tell anyone what is going on for us.

"We don't air our dirty laundry" is the ethos of our family.

I eat because I am stressed and overwhelmed and I feel so isolated.

I eat to drown out the sounds of my parents arguing, my dad yelling, and my mum crying.

I don't want to be poor anymore.

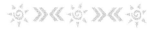

I go with Mum to see the Dean of my college. We can no longer afford the school fees and so I'm going to have to transfer to a public school.

He is kind and understanding as Mum explains our financial situation.

"We would never want to disrupt Suzanne part way through her college education," He begins. "She is a model student with a bright future, so we are offering her a full financial scholarship for the rest of her time here."

Mum and I both burst into tears simultaneously.

"I won't let you down," I say, unsure of whether I am talking to Mum or the Dean.

I decide I want to go to University and become a doctor. Doctors get paid heaps, and I am smart.

Talking with the career advisor I discover I have done the wrong maths subjects for medical school. In order to qualify I need level two maths and not the applied maths that I have completed.

I can attempt level two maths in year 12, however I need permission from that Maths coordinator as I will be skipping level one maths and going straight to level two.

I go to see her but she won't sign off on it.

Frustrated, I go above her to the Dean of the school.

He says he will sign off on it, but it would be better if she did.

I take the form back to her and she looks me in the eye and says, "I will sign this, but I assure you, you will fail" as she begrudgingly signs the form.

I work my ass off for the rest of year 12, and at the end of the year get almost straight A's in level two maths.

I photocopy my report and post it to the Maths coordinator. No one tells me I will fail. I am pissed off about that one B.

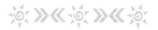

I stand on the scale and see 96 kilograms. I am the biggest I have ever been.

The course load required for year 12 was exhausting, the stress at home from the bankruptcy was hard, and I have no one to talk to as I wasn't allowed to tell anyone.

It's all good though. I am going to be a doctor and make boatloads of money and everything will be fine.

Chapter Five

MEDICAL SCHOOL
2002

I start medical school having been one of the smartest kids in my college.

Although I am used to hard work, having studied hard in school, the course load is gruelling. I have 36 contact hours of classes, labs and tutorials each week, plus the commute time as I live over 40 minutes from campus.

But by far the biggest issue is that I assumed everyone would be studious and focused like me.

They're not.

It's a whole new world of rich people, with snobby parents and a stuck up attitude.

"My daddy bought me a Saab," says Carol one day.

"What's a Saab?" I ask, honestly curious.

"You're not serious?" she laughs dismissively.

"My daddy is the head of neurosurgery at blah hospital," insists someone else. Followed by, "We spend our winters in Hawaii so we never have to be cold; we live in eternal summer."

It's all about who knows who, and I am introduced to the concept of 'it's not what you know, it's who you know'.

My dad's good friend Geoffrey Wells is a guest lecturer; he calls on me because I am the only one he knows.

He makes some backhand comment about knowing my dad and for the first time I am 'in' with the cool crowd.

"What field is your dad in?" someone asks, assuming he is a doctor.

"He's a mini-lab operator," I reply and they nod knowingly and say "ahhh he's in radiology then".

I am never one for false pretenses. "No. He prints photographs."

They give me a look like I am daft. "We know what radiology is, darling."

I laugh. "Not radiology. One hour photos." I walk off.

I want people to like me for me, and not for what they assume my dad does.

I don't really enjoy medical school at all.

I tell my parents every night, "I don't fit in, and I don't enjoy the study."

"Just stick with it." They insist. "It will get better."

I begrudgingly oblige.

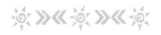

I'm staying at my sister Claudia's house and using her husband's computer, waiting for my first semester results to load, when I see a random orange flashing at the bottom left of the screen.

I ignore it.

A few moments later it starts again.

Frustrated, I click on it, hoping to close whatever it is so I can continue stress eating while madly hitting refresh and hoping that my life isn't over from having failed the first semester.

I see a message. "Hey Mal, have you got the report on the spillage at Tarraleah?"

Gahhhh some work shit. I will just ignore it.

I continue munching and watching the screen.

Next minute the flashing starts again.

Another message. "I really need that report so I can get my response off to Glen."

Mother fucker. I guess I better respond to this. I have no idea what to say.

"Hi, This is Suzanne, Mal's sister-in-law. I'm just borrowing his computer, and will pass on your message when he gets back."

There. Sounds profesh. I hate people'ing.

"Thanks Suzanne. How is Uni going?"

So this random person knows of me. Not awkward at all.

"Fine thanks. Who is this?"

"Jeremy. I work with Mal. He tells me you're studying Japanese," comes the reply.

A requirement for first year Medical school is an un-related elective. I chose Japanese as I had studied it all through school.

We continue chatting about Japan, anime, manga, and other things.

Blissfully, it takes my attention away from contem-plating my career cleaning toilets after my inevitable uni failure while power munching my way through my sis-ter's chocolate stash.

It turns out the platform I'm typing on is called MSN, and Mal has left his account logged in.

After we finish up our conversation, I create my own MSN account and send Jeremy a contact request.

Then I remember my uni results and go check them again, I hold my breath as the screen loads -

Distinction,

Distinction,

High Distinction,

High Distinction.

I survived!

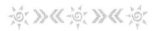

I chat to Jeremy almost every night on MSN.

I ascertain that he is 24 and single.

Too old for me, according to my Mum.

A couple of times he suggests we meet in person.

Nope. Not going to happen.

I'm the biggest I've ever been. 98 kilograms. Once he meets me he won't want to chat to me anymore.

The more we talk the more I do want to meet him though.

I just need to drop a few kilograms fast.

Mum suggests this soup diet she has heard of.

Together we go to the supermarket and buy more vegetables than I would normally eat in a month.

We spend the evening washing, peeling, chopping and cooking.

The soup doesn't taste half bad.

On day one.

A week later I never ever want to touch the soup again. I step on the scales to discover I've dropped 4.5 kilograms.

The soup stays.

Over the following six weeks I lose a total of twelve kilograms and concede to meet Jeremy in person, weighing 86 kilograms.

I have absolutely nothing to wear, and not a lot of money to spend on clothes, so my sister and I go op-shopping.

We find a presentable pair of jeans and a jacket for only $6 for the pair.

She invites Jeremy over to her place for dinner.

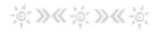

The night arrives, and I'm regretting the jacket because it's too short and doesn't cover my butt.

"You look fine." My sister admonishes for like the fifth time.

When Jeremy arrives there is an awkward stilted greeting, and almost silence during dinner.

For two people who could chat for hours on MSN we have almost nothing to say in person.

Once the dinner is cleared away Claudia leaves the room and comes back brandishing a box. "Let's play Monopoly" she cries.

Well it's not like this night can get any worse.

The game begins and I can't reach the other side of the board so whenever I roll Jeremy will often move my game piece.

About twenty minutes into the game when the stakes are getting high and everyone is strategising, I roll the dice and lean across the table to grab my token.

"Oh so you are capable of moving your own piece?" Jeremy teases with a sparkle on his eye.

Without thinking, I punch him.

He laughs.

The ice is broken, and we finally start to talk.

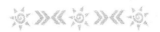

A month later Jeremy and I officially start dating.

A year after that we get engaged.

A year after that we move in together.

Chapter Six

2005

It's my fourth year of medical school, and I am turning 21.

I organise a small gathering at my parents' place as I am not one for big parties. I invite a few of my closest friends.

We talk about our plans for the year.

In semester 2 of your 4th year of medical school you get to choose either a 6 month placement, usually at some exotic location or an honours project.

Given our limited funds, I can't afford a placement, and so I choose to do an honours project.

To make my parents feel better I tell them I prefer honours because it will look better on my academic transcript.

But the truth is I envy my classmates who get to go overseas and experience medicine in other cultures.

The following week Dad proudly presents me with the photos from my 21st birthday party.

I flip through the pile smiling until I come across a picture of me. I barely recognise myself. I am HUGE!

I am wearing a purple shirt striped with silver that I absolutely love and had thought made me look amazing.

Looking at the photos I realise that it doesn't do anything for me except highlight how big I truly am. My best friend standing next to me in the photo is barely visible, being crowded out by my giant bulk.

I immediately burst into tears.

How have I let myself get this big?

When did this happen?

How can I be a doctor when I can't even look after myself?

Who is going to want to see me for medical advice?

They will think I am a big, fat fraud.

I cry uncontrollably. I don't know what to do. I know I need to do something but I don't know what.

I decide it's time to address my weight in a more structured manner.

I research diets online and eventually decide on Weight Watchers.

I have kind of done it before when I was a kid and my Mum used to go to meetings. But I haven't officially done it myself.

I decide that this is the approach for me.

I call my Mum and ask if she wants to join with me. She agrees.

I officially join Weight Watchers with my mum.

I am SO excited to finally be doing something about my weight.

This time it's going to be different because I am committed.

I am going to go to meetings every week and get weighed in and do this officially.

The night of the first meeting I am very nervous.

I haven't weighed myself in months. I have NO idea what I weigh.

But I also have a feeling of quiet determination. My wait is over. I am finally ready to address this once and for all.

With trepidation I join the queue for the scales.

I am having flashbacks to my grade 3 poster experience and thinking everyone is going to laugh at me.

I consider bolting for the door and calling this whole thing off.

The thought must be written all over my face as the leader approaches me and asks how I am going.

She assures me that everything here is confidential, and I can share as much or as little as I like. Feeling reassured I continue to stand in line and await my fate on the scales.

I get to the front of the queue, and I am pleasantly surprised to see that the scales are set up so only the person weighing you in can see the number.

For some reason I had mentally envisioned it being blazoned around the room for everyone to see. Plus the lady doing the weighing in is easily as big as I am, if not bigger.

SUZANNE CULBERG

I am equal parts excited to not be the fattest person in the room, and questioning whether this program will really work, given the staff also have weight issues.

I push these thoughts out of my mind and step on the scale.

I can't see the number, but the weigher dutifully records it in my record book and discreetly closes the cover and passes it to me.

I open it up and stop in my tracks 120.3kg.

No way!

I feel the urge to vomit.

I knew I was over the 100kg mark but 120.3kg!

Holy hell.

I fight the urge to run from the room and do a Maccas drive thru run.

How has it come to this?

According to the record book I am trying to read without anyone looking over my shoulder, I need to lose 52kg to be considered healthy. 52!

My best friend doesn't even weigh that much!

I need to lose a whole person?!

My urge to quit before I even start is strong.

The leader once again materialises beside me. Perhaps she could sense my impending bolt, and she gently touches me on the arm. "This is the last time you will see that number. It's just a starting point. You are here for a reason. Remember that and let's go and take a seat and get started."

I follow her blindly and sit down, trying to discreetly wipe away the tears that have gathered in my eyes.

I listen with rapt attention to the meeting; I even take notes.

At the end of the meeting I go and buy all the things. The points guide, eating out guide, exercise guide, tracker, cookbooks, snacks, I buy the lot.

Lord knows how I am going to afford this.

But once I make a commitment I am ALL in.

I go home, and I pour over it all.

I stay up for hours planning my meals, planning my exercise, working out the best points for my buck.

The very next day I go back to Oceana, the very same gym I had joined in high school, and I sign up.

I also join the hospital gym.

Ever the over achiever I figure two gym memberships are better than one.

I love Oceana for the pool and the group fitness classes.

But the hospital gym is so convenient as I can attend before I start my rounds or during my lunch break.

This is it.

In my first week I lose 2.3kg.

In my second 1.6kg.

By my third week I earn my 5kg star. I have totally got this. I am on a roll.

I rack up rewards like there's no tomorrow.

5kg, 5% loss, 10kg, 10% loss, 15kg.

I feel unstoppable.

I count my points, and I do my exercise consistently.

But the more weight I drop, the less points I can eat, and I find this a real struggle.

Especially because the lighter and fitter I become, the more exercise I do. So I feel hungry more often.

I am a stickler for the rules, and my Weight Watchers manual says I can eat NO more than 4 exercise points per day, even though I am earning up to 20 exercise points.

I struggle because some days I am really truly hungry and other days I am not.

Some days I eat my allocation of points before lunch, and then I am trying to get through the rest of the day on points-free foods like celery and clear soup.

Other days, it's 8pm and I haven't eaten anywhere near my points allocation and so I am eating junk to increase my points.

It's made very clear to us that we are not to eat above or below our points allocation by more than 2 points on any given day.

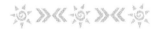

2006

I return to University for my 5th year of medical school.

Everyone is back from their placement or their honours project, and the majority of the class haven't seen me in over 6 months.

Some people don't even recognise me. Introducing themselves to me as if I am a new student.

Each year the medical student society publishes a yearbook. Having never been a party girl I have never shown an interest in buying it, I doubt I would even make the cut.

I go to the library, and I overhear some people snickering and whispering about me.

They run off when I approach, and I notice they have dropped the year book. I pick it up and see a picture of me from 3rd year. We had had a 'halfway graduation' party complete with a massive cake.

Someone had snapped a picture of me next to the cake. In the 'before' picture there was me standing next to the cake, with a thought bubble saying "Me so hungry" and in the 'after' picture someone had photoshopped out the cake and the thought bubble said "better now".

I feel my stomach churn.

I keep flipping through the book.

On one of the following pages is a series of 'quotes' from students.

There was one attributed to me saying "I used to eat one mars bar and drink one can of coke per day, but now that I go to the gym I can have two mars bars a day and two cans of coke".

My hands start to shake and I can feel the rash of despair rising up as my face gets really hot.

I have never felt more hurt and humiliated.

I have been teased my entire life, and I have put up with it, but enough is enough.

I see red.

These people aren't just any schoolyard bullies, they are going to be doctors.

If they treat me like this, how are they going to treat their future patients?

I grab the book and storm off to find the year coordinator.

I take the book right out of the library, not caring that I set off the sensors because I haven't borrowed it officially, I just keep on marching.

I storm into Mr Lester's office, not even bothering to knock, and I slap that book down on his desk.

He looks up at me in shock and before he even has the chance to question me, I pick the book back up and wave it in his face "Have you seen this?" I ask, before bursting into tears.

Mr Lester is a kind and caring coordinator. He passes me a box of tissues and does his best to console me.

He tells me to leave it with him.

The following week the two students responsible sidle up to me after a lecture.

They give me some weak assed apology, telling me they are sorry that my feelings are hurt.

Nothing screams 'fake apology' like someone saying they are sorry you feel hurt.

Talk about taking no ownership about what they had done.

What was I expecting?

I take the matter further. I send emails to the head of TUMMS (the medical student society) and to the Dean.

I hear nothing back.

It seems bullying at medical school is the same as bullying at any other school I have been to, swept under the carpet and ignored.

I spend some time really contemplating my future.

All I really ever want to do is help people, as cliche as that sounds. I thought I could do that by being a doctor, but it seems doctors aren't immune to bullying.

I weigh 77 kilograms now, less than 10 kilograms from my goal. My absolute favourite thing to do, what lights me up each day, is going to the gym.

I love my classes, and I love the supportive environment of the gym.

I don't like medical school at all. The hours suck, and that isn't going to get better any time soon.

The workload is enormous. I am not afraid of hard work, but the content is so dry. It feels like a hard slog to keep up with all the reading, tutorials and prac classes.

I speak to my friends and family about quitting. They all encourage me to stay, "You are so close to graduating," they say, "only 18 months to go."

What they don't realise is when you graduate from medical school you are basically a doctor of nothing. You still have your intern year, then your residency, then your registrar training to go. It's the better part of ten years before you're finally finished.

Even then you aren't done, you are never done training to be a doctor, as you have to keep up all your skills and continuous education, as well as research and write papers and publish.

The thought of this life laid out in front of me makes me want to scream.

What if I want to have kids?

What if I want to just do nothing at the end of the day?

I decide enough is enough, and I quit medical school.

I don't want this life.

There are a myriad of reasons I leave medical school. But one of the biggest ones is that my trust is well and truly broken.

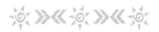

Now that my entire future plan has been thrown out the window, I contemplate what I want to do with my life.

I want to help fat people lose weight and live the life they've always dreamed.

So I train as a gym instructor and personal trainer.

I undertake my certificate three and four simultaneously. Thanks to my medical school background I receive recognition of prior learning for the anatomy and physiology units.

The day after I complete my certifications I start work at the gym.

My career has finally begun.

Within the first week I am booked out as a personal trainer, having 77 clients sign up.

I do have the advantage of their having witnessed my weight transformation over the past year.

Jeremy and I buy our first apartment, get married and make plans for our future.

Chapter Seven

My new career soon shows its limitations.

I have no boundaries, and I don't want to let anyone down, so I book clients whenever they want a session.

I have no self-care, and my own workouts go on the backburner.

Being a PT, I work when other people don't, so I am at the gym every weekday from 6am till about 11am, then I come home for lunch, only to restart at about 3pm and work through till 9pm.

I put my needs last, often not eating properly, and when I do eat it's a grab and run.

I start to eat chocolate again, and more and more of it.

I think back to those snide remarks in the medical school year book about eating 2 mars bars a day, and I don't care, I do it anyway.

I can feel the weight creeping back on.

I've regained about 15kg and no one has noticed but me. It's amazing what you can get away with when you live in track pants.

I am saved from having to face this weight gain by a move to Queensland. Jeremy gets a job offer we can't refuse, and we set off to the mainland, planning to stay for one year and then return to Tasmania.

I assure myself that once we have moved and settled in Queensland I will get back on track, lose the 15kg and everything will be fine again.

We move to Kingaroy, a small town in South East Queensland with two very small gyms.

I approach both to ask for work, but neither are hiring at the moment.

I weigh 92 kilos. I feel it's my weight that is holding me back, they probably don't want to hire a fat personal trainer.

I have gone from being a 'celebrity' at my local gym where everyone has seen me transform, to a fat person trying desperately to hold on to a fit person's body.

I join both gyms as a member. I'm desperate to reclaim my former figure. I have worked so hard, and I can feel it slipping away.

I don't like either gym, to be honest. In Tasmania I had been a member of Oceana which I went to since school and later Feminine Lines which is female only fitness, and I felt more comfortable in those gyms.

Here I feel like I stand out because I am not local and because I am big. I just don't gel with the place.

Belonging is a VERY important thing for me. Beyond merely fitting in, belonging means I am free to be myself.

Fitting in always feels like I have to try hard to be someone I am not.

I feel like I neither belong nor fit in, and I use it as an excuse not to attend regularly.

I don't have a job, and I feel like I am biding my time. As we only plan to live in Kingaroy for one year I don't really make an effort to go out and meet people. I am not overly social anyway.

I stay home, and I watch DVDs, bingeing ALL the shows that I didn't get to watch while I was studying at medical school.

I have never really had a chance to just relax before, I have spent my life either studying or working and so it's a welcome relief to just sit back and do nothing.

It's not long before I am bored.

When I get bored I eat.

I often find myself absentmindedly standing at the fridge or cupboard, staring at the contents.

Eating gives me something to do.

Eating is important.

Despite telling myself I am enjoying the isolation, in truth I am very lonely and food is my friend.

Food is always there.

Food never has nasty things to say.

Food doesn't judge or bully.

Food is whatever I need it to be. I have spent the better part of the last two years dieting my ass off, literally, and I am sick of it.

I keep telling myself I will start again tomorrow.

Tomorrow will be different.

Tomorrow I won't eat chocolate.
Tomorrow I will go back to the gym.
Tomorrow I will make better food choices.
I'll definitely start tomorrow.

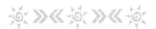

The new year starts. It's 2008. This is going to be my year.

New Year. New you. I tell myself this over and over as I create a vision board, madly cutting and pasting pictures onto a giant poster. Just looking at all the cute outfits I dream of wearing and wonderful holidays I want to take inspires me into action.

I start looking for a new diet. One that will work with my new resolve and willpower.

I see an ad for Tony Ferguson, and the before and after photos convince me.

There is no pharmacy nearby that sells it, so I have to drive all the way to Toowoomba to buy it.

Driving is a big anxiety for me, I had a car accident two days before we left Tasmania, and I've avoided driving as much as possible since.

As scared as I am to drive all the way to Toowoomba, I am more scared of being fat, so off I go.

I make an appointment to speak with the consultant. She weighs me and takes my measurements.

I weigh 117kg.

SHIT!

How did this happen?

I want to cry. I am almost back to my starting weight before Weight Watchers.

The lady rattles on with a list of all the things I can't have. One of them is diet coke.

"What do you mean I can't have diet coke?" I cry out. I love soft drink.

Switching from regular coke to diet coke was the one habit I have maintained since Weight Watchers.

I loved how diet coke was zero points in Weight Watchers so I could drink as much as I liked.

I am tempted to leave.

I stand up, and say to the lady "I don't think this is the program for me" and go to walk out the door.

"You can have caffeine free diet coke," she says.

I pause in the doorway.

"Ok" I say.

I spend a small fortune on Tony Ferguson products.

Reminiscent of my Weight Watchers days I am not someone who does things by half measures; when I am in, I'm in.

I buy every flavour of shake and soup and bar. I buy the cookbooks. I find the list of allowable foods, and I go to the supermarket on the way home and buy everything from that list.

According to the plan I am to have a shake for breakfast, a shake or soup or bar for lunch and then a regular meal for dinner. With NO starchy carbs. But apparently I can make no-tatoes, which is basically mashed potato substituted with cauliflower.

I start the very next morning.

Good lord the shake tastes revolting.

I really question what on Earth it is that I am doing.

Perhaps the soups are better. I try one of those at lunch and nearly gag. I manage to choke it down.

By dinner time I am absolutely starving. I don't feel like the shake or soup did anything to curb my appetite.

I make the no-tatoes and am bitterly disappointed, they taste ghastly.

No-tatoes? Well they got the name right because they certainly aren't potatoes.

My resolve is beginning to waiver, and it's only day one.

I manage to survive my first week.

I drive out to Toowoomba to be weighed in. I tentatively step on the scales.

110kg.

That can't be right.

I step off and on again.

It still reads 110kg. I do the numbers in my head. 7 kilograms.

I jump off the scales and run around the room squealing.

I hug the consultant. I grab my phone and ring Jeremy.

"I've lost 7 kilograms!" I shout. "7 in only 1 week!"

I have never had a result like this. I feel a renewed sense of commitment.

I drive home excited by the upcoming week.

I do everything the same, and I return the following week and excitedly step on the scales.

109.9kg.

This can't be right?

100 grams. I have lost a measly 100 grams!

What the fuck?

I have suffered through these horrible soups, these disgusting shakes and these cardboard tasting bars for only 100 bloody grams.

I could pee a bigger number than this.

I storm out of the chemist, with the poor consultant calling after me, and march myself into the nearest Coles supermarket. I go immediately to the confectionary aisle, and snatch up a block of Blackforest chocolate. As I'm walking out of the aisle, I pause and return and grab a block of Topdeck too.

"Why not? 100 bloody grams," I mutter to myself dejectedly.

I also grab a tin of condensed milk.

Might as well, all the good stuff hasn't gotten me anywhere.

I finish the black forest chocolate before I even make it back to the car.

An entire block demolished in a matter of minutes.

I eat the Topdeck on the drive home.

I am miserable.

When I get home I put the condensed milk in the fridge to get cold. Then I go sit on the couch, feeling sorry for myself, and swear off Tony Ferguson.

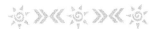

We've been living in Kingaroy for over six months, and I am bored. I feel like all I do is sit at home all day waiting for Jeremy to come back from work. I'm not used to having nothing to do, and although I've enjoyed bingeing TV shows, I've reached a point where I am just done.

I can't go back to personal training, I am too big and too unfit.

I am not sure what to do for work as my Bachelor of Medical Science, although a degree, doesn't open up any clear job prospects.

So I decide to go back to university to get a graduate diploma in teaching. I find an online course that runs for twelve months and enrol.

The reading material is very dry, and I struggle to wade my way through it. I have never enjoyed humanities subjects. I much prefer maths and science-based study.

I start to eat a lot of junk food, telling myself that the sugar helps the information stick. I really struggle to commit to the workload because it's boring and it doesn't hold my attention at all.

The first half of the semester is purely theory work. Lots of reading and assignments.

The second half of the semester looks more promising as we get to have practical placements in a local school.

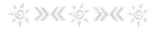

"I have nothing to wear!" I yell down the phone to my Mum, as I frantically throw clothes around my wardrobe.

"What do you mean you have nothing to wear?" she calmly replies. "What about that nice pin-striped shirt, or the emerald one or the purple one?"

"They don't fit!" I exclaim "Nothing fits!"

"How much weight have you gained?" she asks.

"I don't know," I moan.

I am secretly too scared to get on the scales.

I am panicking because I have NOTHING to wear, and my school placement is starting in a week.

I fire up my laptop and hurriedly google "fastest way to lose weight" and am blown away by the pages and pages of results.

The options are overwhelming.

I open each page in a new tab, scrolling each before dismissing it and moving on to my next option.

I finally choose Body Trim.

It looks fairly simple. For the first 3 days you "detox" and eat nothing but protein, so I had better start immediately before my School placement begins.

I clean out the kitchen pantry and fridge of all the 'bad' foods.

I am an old hat at this by now.

I put everything on the bench and have a last 'hurrah' eating ALL the things I won't be allowed to eat from tomorrow.

I say to myself *This is the last time,* and I congratulate myself on how amazing I am going to look.

I then go to the supermarket and stock up on all things protein, corned beef, chicken, tuna.

I am ready to go.

The next morning I take a deep breath before I weigh in, ready to see my new starting weight.

Tentatively I step on the scales.

130 kilograms!

Holy shit!

I am officially the fattest I have ever been.

With grim determination I commit to this Body Trim program.

I head into the kitchen and grab my 100 grams of chicken breast for breakfast.

It feels weird eating meat for breakfast.

I have always been a toast or cereal eater. But hey, it's only three days. How hard can it be?

By morning tea time I am quite hungry, so I eagerly drain my tin of tuna in springwater.

It tastes so bland. I remember why I can't stand fish, it's the horrible texture it has.

For lunch I dutifully weigh out my next 100 grams of chicken breast. I still feel hungry after this but I push on. I tell myself *I can do this.*

At afternoon tea I inhale my next tin of tuna, not even minding the texture.

By dinner time I am really quite hungry, but I am also determined, so I measure out my serve of beef and eat it slowly, trying to savour the taste.

I am still hungry after dinner and so I go to bed early to stave off the hunger pains.

I wake up the next morning feeling totally flat.

I feel like my brain is foggy, and I can't concentrate.

By morning tea time my head has started to ache; it's so bad that I can't even think.

I log on to the Body Trim forums and explain my symptoms and am re-assured that this is perfectly normal.

Apparently the blinding headache is a combination of sugar and caffeine withdrawals and my body going into ketosis from the low carbohydrate.

I have tried a lot of diets in my time, but I have NEVER felt like this.

I literally want to die.

I draw the blinds closed and curl up in bed.

The people on the forums promise me that this feeling will pass, and so I try to sleep and hope they are right.

Day three is by far the hardest day.

I am sick of chicken.

I am sick of tuna.

I am sick of beef.

All I want is a piece of bloody bread.

I have never before craved bread in my life. This feels like torture.

I remind myself that I have never known true torture. I am a fortunate person living in a first world country, and I have done this to myself.

This is all my fault because I can't control myself around food.

I am a fat failure, with no one to blame but myself.

Day four dawns and I am so excited I rush to the scales to see the result of my detox.

126 kilograms! I've lost 4 kilograms in 3 days.

How bloody marvellous.

It's time to move to the next phase.

For phase 2 of Body Trim, I am excited to be allowed to eat something other than meat. But the list is pretty restrictive.

A protein serving is no more than 100 grams. Which really doesn't look like much.

On the bright side I can have 'unlimited' vegetables as long as they come from the list, which excludes potatoes, peas and corn which are my favourites.

According to the plan I am to eat six times per day, with no more than three hours between meals.

This seems like a lot to me.

On day four I eat:

Breakfast- Egg white omelette with onions, spinach and ricotta

Snack- Low fat cottage cheese

Lunch- Tuna with lettuce, tomatoes, alfalfa sprouts and onions.

Snack- Chickpeas

Dinner- Lentil and Spinach Soup

Snack — can't do it! Don't like eating in the evening, unless it's chocolate or ice-cream, which of course are strictly forbidden.

On day ten, having lost a total of six kilograms, I quit body trim.

I just want some bloody weetbix, or a piece of toast.

I feel like I am slowly dying, eating like this, so I decide to just do my own thing.

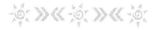

I walk to and from my school placement.

I cook meals every evening and take the leftovers to school the following day for lunch.

I go to the gym three to five times per week.

This becomes my routine.

Over the following four months I lose twenty kilograms.

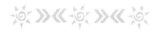

I don't enjoy teaching.

Although the hours are great, the work expected outside school hours is higher than I anticipated.

Lesson planning is especially arduous.

I tell myself this will get easier once I have had a few years under my belt, as I can recycle the lesson plans from year to year.

I persevere.

I complete semester one of my teaching diploma and score high distinctions in every subject.

I am very proud of myself. I know how to be a model student.

Unfortunately the same can't be said of my own students.

I get frustrated for all the hours I spend diligently creating lesson plans, only to take them to school and receive total disinterest from the students.

"Don't you know how many hours I spent planning this? Why aren't you grateful?" I want to scream.

The day comes for my first set of parent-teacher interviews. I am excited to finally speak to some of the parents and see how I can better help their children engage and learn.

I sit down after school. I am almost wriggling in my chair because I am so excited for this opportunity.

Rosella Parker is the first parent who is coming in. Austin's mum.

I have a momentary freak out. *What do I call her? Mrs Parker?* Sounds too formal. *Rosella?* it feels weird to call her by her first name, too grown up.

I was only a student last year and don't feel ready for speaking to adults on a first name basis.

For God's sake woman you are a grown up.

I can feel my palms start to sweat and the rash of despair creeping up my neck and cheeks.

I look at my watch, still undecided. The time is up. I have to go and get her now.

I walk out to the waiting room. There are so many parents there. I feel a bit daunted.

"Ros-eee-ella?" I call out.

Moron, you can't even say her name right, how on Earth does she think you are able to teach her kid?

A lady stands up from the crowd and walks toward me. I smile, well I try to smile, it feels more like a wince.

"This way," I say and lead her to the interview room.

"What do you call this?" she demands, waving a report at me before I have even closed the door.

"P-pardon?" I stammer.

"You gave Austin all C's."

I frown. This is not what I expected.

"Cccccccccccc-s" she repeats, drawing out the letter, as if I didn't understand it the first time.

I am a bit flustered, and am unsure how to direct this conversation. I assumed she knew her son never completed his homework and was often disinterested, even disruptive in class.

"Well..." I begin, stalling for time as my brain madly tries to come up with a delicate way to have this conversation. "Austin very rarely submits his assignments on time and his last few tests have not been completed..."

She cuts me off.

"Do you know how hard it is to be a teenager these days? There are so many responsibilities. Austin wants to be a vet you know. He's going to need much better grades than this to get into University. So you're going to fix this, right?"

I am flabbergasted.

She wants me to fix this?

Hard to be a teenager these days?

Lady, it wasn't that long ago I was a teenager myself.

Vet school with his grades? Who is she kidding? I just came out of medical school and you needed straight A's for that. Vet school is even harder.

I fumble my way through the rest of the conversation.

As I say goodbye to Rosella I think to myself *Oh well, there's bound to be one in every bunch, I am sure the rest of the interviews will go well.*

I am wrong.

Many of the other interviews follow a similar pattern. Each parent questioning their child's grades and implying, sometimes indirectly but very often rather pointedly, that it is my fault that their child isn't achieving.

They take no personal responsibility, like it is totally up to me what their child achieves, or doesn't.

Reflecting back on my own efforts in year twelve, and the amount of work I put in to achieve the grades I did, I begin to question whether teaching is right for me.

The interviews drone on well into the evening.

When they finally finish I drag myself wearily to the car.

Arriving home, I boot up the computer and go searching for jobs.

I find a job listing for my local medicare office. The salary is more than I will get for teaching, and the hours look really reasonable.

I tidy up my resume and submit it.

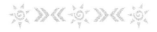

It's a relief to quit teaching. It was a lot more work than I anticipated for very little reward.

I begin my job at medicare with real excitement. The pay is excellent, the hours are awesome, and outside of work hours I don't need to think about work at all.

At medical school, outside of course hours I had to study continuously.

While working at the gym, outside of personal training sessions and group fitness classes, I had to learn choreography and respond to client text messages.

Being a student teacher, outside of classes I had to do lesson planning and marking.

I feel like I have never had true 'down time' before, except for the period between being a personal trainer and starting teaching, when although I had freedom, I soon got bored.

This medicare job feels like an awesome balance.

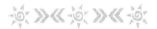

I arrive home from work and dump all the groceries on the bench.

I flop down on the couch and flip on the television.

I will just watch five minutes of this show, and then I will cook dinner.

Five minutes becomes an episode, and so the window of time I had created for going to the gym disappears.

I walk into the kitchen and open the fridge, as I begin to pull out ingredients I yawn.

Cooking seems like such an effort.

It's been a big day, so many cranky customers. I will order pizza just this once, and I will go back to the gym and the healthy eating tomorrow.

Chapter Eight

My work pants don't fit.
Not even remotely.

I get away with not doing them up, because my long shirt covers them and no one can see. But I can feel my stomach protruding over the top whenever I sit down.

They are so tight they leave marks on my hips and there is now only one pair of work trousers and one shirt that I can just barely squeeze into.

The one shirt, although long enough to hide the fact that my trousers don't do up, hugs every fat roll around my middle and strains at my bust.

I worry one day I will pop a button and hit a customer in the eye.

I hope when it eventually happens it's at least a difficult customer. It might serve them right.

I have to go home and wash my uniform every night because nothing else fits, and Queensland is bloody hot.

Uniform allotment at work isn't for another few months, and I don't think they make a bigger size than this.

I have never felt this low.

I flip through my wedding album, looking at pictures from what seems like forever ago, but it wasn't even two years, and I realise I am literally twice the woman I used to be.

I'm sobbing.

I feel like such a failure with no one to blame but myself. I'm the fat fuck who can't control herself around food.

I can't share my feelings with anyone. No one from back home in Tasmania knows just how much weight I have gained because I haven't been home in over a year.

I worry I won't fit in a plane seat anymore, so I couldn't go home even if I wanted to.

I haven't made any friends in Kingaroy. My work colleagues, although friendly, aren't the same as friends.

I feel so isolated.

I scroll online, looking for inspiration, searching for the answer, the thing that is going to fix me.

I am so sick of this cycle.

With every new diet I come across online I ask myself *Is this going to be just another weight loss thing I spend money on that doesn't do anything?*

I decide to go back to Weight Watchers.

I have had great success with that in the past. I know it works, when I do the work.

I walk into the Monday night Weight Watchers meeting and have a sense of total deja vu. I sit down at the newbies table. A glowing leader approaches.

Where on Earth do they get these perky people?

"Welcome to Weight Watchers, my name is Lyn. Is this your first time?" she says.

In a different context that sentence could be oh so wrong lady.

"Hi, I'm Suzanne, and this is my fourth attempt," I reply thinking about the other times I'd tried Weight Watchers over the years.

I feel like I am at AA. Hi, my name is Suzanne, and I am a food-aholic.

I listen to the same spiel I have heard three times previously.

The points system has been slightly revised, but the premise is the same.

Before I know it, it's time to weigh in.

I drag out my chair and slowly stand, as if by dragging this moment out I will somehow weigh less. I join the back of the queue.

I know I am the biggest I have ever been.

Will these scales even weigh me?

I wonder if anyone has ever been too big to be weighed in. What do they do then?

As if sensing my impending flee, Lyn comes over and grabs my arm.

"No need to queue darling, because this is your first week you get to go straight to the front."

Great.

Thanks, Lyn. Good to know all Weight Watchers leaders are equally helpful.

I hand over my card, and step on the scale. I look down, no point delaying the inevitable.

144.6kg! Holy fuck.

My legs tremble. The room starts to spin. I hurriedly snatch the card from the weigher and stumble to the nearest chair and collapse into it. It shudders under my weight.

I can imagine the headline.

'Woman breaks chair at Weight Watchers'

The meeting begins, but I don't hear a word. At one stage everyone turns to me, so I gather I am being introduced. I smile dumbly and manage an awkward wave.

I want to go home. Not to the stupid house we are renting in Kingaroy.

Home to my family.

I can't go home, even though I long to. No one would recognise me now. I am literally twice the person I was when I left. It hasn't even been 3 years, and I have doubled my body weight. How did this happen?

How am I here again?

I resist the urge to do a drive thru run and head straight home after the meeting.

I sit at the kitchen table with all the books I have bought from Weight Watchers, and once again I commit to getting this done.

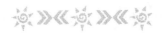

I diligently follow Weight Watchers eating guidelines for the next three months, and I drop twenty kilograms.

People are finally starting to notice. I feel pretty good about myself and am ready to commence exercising again.

A new high-end personal training studio has opened in town. It is expensive, but I decide to invest. I hesitantly hand over my credit card, and sign up for three sessions per week.

A perky girl with blond hair and big boobs bounds over to me "Hi, I'm Brooke," she says. "I am so excited to be your trainer. You must be Suzanne."

Great, I am being trained by Barbie. How old is she anyway? She looks like a kid.

"Let's start on the treadmill," says Barbie.

"Sure," I reply, trying to smile, but hiding a grimace.

"You press this button to start it, this button to pause. Be sure to attach this clip to your shirt, it's the emergency stop button…." She drones on, and I try to look like I am listening.

Does she treat everyone like this? Or does she assume that because I am fat I also don't know the basics of a treadmill?

I long to tell her I am an ex-personal trainer. But I am too mortified to speak up. Personal trainers don't allow themselves to get like this.

I debate leaving.

Barbie must sense my boredom. Because she smiles at me and says, "Let's step this up a bit, ok?"

We move from the treadmill to the cross trainer.

This is more like it.

I continue to see Barbie three times per week, and my fitness improves at a rapid rate. I guess that old story about muscle memory really has some merit.

One Thursday morning I turn up for my 6am session.

"Want to try a new challenge today?" asks Barbie.

"Bring it," I respond.

"Box jumps are in the house!" she sings excitedly.

I am immediately unsure.

Jumps are totally not my thing. I have flashbacks to high jump attempts at school, and how I would feign just about any illness to get out of them.

"I really don't know. I am a bit hesistant to…" I begin.

"How much do you want to lose this spare tyre?" asks Barbie, poking me in the belly.

"More than anything," I reply.

"Well box jumps are a calorie killer," she insists.

I follow her across the studio and watch as she executes a perfect box jump.

Watching her do this and imagining myself doing this, I am immediately reminded of those memes "what I think I look like when I plank versus what I actually look like" and I wonder to myself if they have memes like that for box jumps.

I stand contemplating the box. I feel a sense of dread and like a deep part of me is trying to tell me not to do this.

"Remind yourself of how much you want to shift this," insists Barbie jabbing me in the belly once more.

So I jump.

As soon as I land I feel the jar from my ankles right through my body to my jaw, and I feel a pain in my hips. My eyes water and my head spins a bit.

"I am not sure about this," I start to say.

"It's always awkward the first time," Barbie says. "You will get used to it."

I continue the session, but the pain intensifies. Even after we cool down and stretch, it's still there.

I go home and shower and it doesn't go away.

I commence work, and all day I feel I am shifting in my chair and can't quite get comfortable.

I take a couple of nurofen tablets and do my best to ignore it.

It's a busy day, and I am exhausted. I go to bed that night and fall straight to sleep.

I wake up on Friday morning, and as soon as I move to roll over I feel pain.

Sharp stabbing pain right down my back.

I can't roll over.

I shuffle my way over to the side of the bed and reach blindly for my phone.

I call my mum.

"You've just put your back out, Suze. There's no need to worry. Take the day off work, and it will get better over the weekend. Remember me putting my back out when you were a kid? A few days rest and you'll be good to go."

I did remember her putting her back out when I was a kid.

I call in sick for work, take some more nurofen, and settle back in bed with some books for the day.

Over the weekend my back doesn't get any better.

I cancel PT sessions for the week, but go back to work on Monday.

For the next two weeks I don't do any exercise. But I do attend work.

My boss encourages me to visit a doctor to get my back checked. I make an appointment for Monday.

The doctor promptly sends me for an X-ray and then a CT scan.

"You have bi-lateral pars fractures at L5-S1," he tells me.

"So what does that mean?" I ask.

"We will start with a prescription for mobic and two weeks of rest and we will see from there," he says.

"Rest? So no gym?" I ask.

He laughs "No gym, no work, no nothing. I mean total rest," he says.

Oh.

I have a sense of dread.

No gym, for two more weeks, for a start. Shit.

I'm going to get fatter.

I follow the doctors orders and for two weeks I pretty much sit on the couch or lie in bed.

I am cleared to return to work, but forbidden to exercise.

I am so worried about regaining weight.

After a few more weeks I am cleared to walk in the pool. I have never been so excited to be able to do something. I join the local pool that day.

I feel so free in the water. As soon as I enter the pool all the pain in my back goes away.

I walk up and down the pool feeling like a free woman. Then as soon as I haul myself up, and my body leaves the water, the pain returns.

I walk laps in the pool for one month.

Then I begin to swim.

I adjust to the pain. It is a constant dull ache in my back that sometimes radiates outward if I move too fast or bend or reach too far.

Despite the pain, I continue to eat well, to move when I can, to diligently attend my Weight Watchers meetings, and the weight continues to drop away.

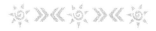

After a few months I attend a local health expo that I see advertised on a local noticeboard.

I am wandering up and down the aisles when I see a sign about back pain.

I stop to grab a brochure and a smiling dark haired woman comes over and introduces herself.

"Hi, I'm Laura. Do you know about chiropractic care?"

I have immediate flashbacks to medical school. Chiropractors aren't spoken well of in medical circles. But she seems friendly and I really don't have anywhere to be, so I decide to chat.

I tell Laura about my back and my weight loss and she is very attentive and seems caring, asking lots of questions.

She gets me to turn my head this way, and that way.

With my permission she then feels my shoulders and back and asks me to walk forward and turn.

She explains to me what she thinks is going on and asks me if I would like to schedule an appointment.

The following week I go to Laura's practise with my x-rays in hand. I watch a DVD about chiropractic care, we review my x-rays together, and I have my first adjustment.

Once she is finished and I stand up, I swear I feel an inch taller.

For the first time in months my back is totally pain free. I hesitantly take a step forward waiting for the return of the pain, but there is nothing.

"Wow. I can't believe the difference I feel. I only have my 'normal' pain now."

Laura raises her eyebrows. "Your normal pain?"

I burst out laughing, and she joins in. I felt an instant connection to her when I met her, and this has been confirmed now.

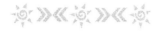

Over an eighteen month period from this round of joining Weight Watchers, through my personal training, my
back injury and my recovery I manage to lose sixty kilograms. I have gone from 144 kilograms to 84 kilograms.
But once I hit the 84 kilogram mark my resolve starts to
wobble.

I skip yet another Weight Watchers meeting.

I don't have time. I will go back next week.

I seem to be having variations of this conversation
with myself over and over.

I get home from work, and I am too tired to cook so
I just eat toast and vegemite for dinner.

One time won't hurt.

I will get more organised again tomorrow.

I can lie to myself so easily. But lying to my friends
is harder. I text Laura, who has become my close friend
and exercise buddy, "Can't come for a run today, feeling
a bit under the weather."

She replies, "Come out anyway babe, the fresh air
might do you good."

Dammit, how am I going to get out of this?

I punch out a quick reply. "Thanks babe but my back
is really twinging today, I think rest is best."

"Come on hun, we can just walk today. Let's pop
into my office for a quick adjustment first. You will feel
better for moving."

I consider telling her the truth. That I am really struggling at the moment.

Everything feels like too much.

I worry about what she will think? She has only known me as the super committed and dedicated Suze. What if she doesn't like the real me?

I can't deal with all these thoughts. I send her a quick text promising I will be back tomorrow, and I raid the freezer for ice cream.

When I am eating I don't have to think.

I can feel my weight creeping up. But I ignore it. I pretty much live in active wear outside of work, and tights can be very forgiving.

I get invited out to the movies and decide to glam up a bit.

I pull out my favourite jeans and go to slide them on and I struggle to get them past my hips.

Shit.

I decide I might as well face the music now, and I do the walk of shame to the bathroom and step on the scales.

I have probably gained about four kilos.

I mentally prepare myself to see the number 88 on the scales.

88 like to fat sailors, wobble wobble, oh the irony.

I step on.

92 kilos!

How did this happen?

I am torn between warring thoughts of....

I've got to do something, stat!

And

Where are the tim tams?

I step off the scale.

I find something else to wear and head out to the movies.

I don't pay any attention to the film. My mind is a constant blur of thoughts.

I could do Tony Ferguson again for a bit, whip these kilos off with some shakes.

Nah, I bloody hated Tony Ferguson.

I could do Body Trim....

I don't even finish that thought. Just the idea of doing the three days of pure protein again is enough to make me nauseous.

My mind is reeling with so many ideas. All the things I had tried in the past, the CSIRO diet, the heart foundation soup diet, the cabbage soup diet.

None of these options sound appealing.

After the movie one of my friends suggests pizza, and so we head to the local pizza place.

I am still distracted by my thoughts and am barely following the conversation. One of them mentions The Biggest Loser and my ears perk up.

They are talking about one of the TV shows trainer's having her own online fitness program. Michelle Bridges 12WBT program.

I start to listen with rapt attention.

12WBT? Why hadn't I thought of that?

I can hardly wait to get home and look it up.

As soon as I find it I spend hours scrolling through all the before and after photos. Admiring all the beautiful women.

I enrol immediately. Perfect timing as the next round is due to start in two weeks. This looks like exactly what I have been wanting. I am so excited, this is going to be 'The Thing'!

I start the warm up work the very next day. I do all of the activities including introducing myself in the forums, taking before photographs, doing a baseline fitness test.

As soon as the meal plans are released I print them off and go shopping for all of the ingredients.

Some of them are bizarre and expensive and then we only use them in one meal.

I am annoyed at the waste and the cost.

I push down my annoyance and persevere, this is going to be 'The Thing' after all.

I find the calorie restriction a challenge.

On Weight Watchers there were a lot of 'points free foods' which we could eat freely without having to measure or track. This is not the case with 12WBT. Every morsel needs to be weighed, measured and accounted for.

1200 calories doesn't seem to go far.

I ignore my reservations about the food and fully dive into the exercise. I love the challenge of burning 500 calories on weekdays and 1000 calories on Saturdays.

My love for exercise is renewed.

But my most favourite part of all is the mindset component.

In all the programs I have tried before none of them have ever even addressed this. It was always "create a calorie deficit with calories in versus calories out." What you think about it wasn't even a factor.

I watch all the mindset videos several times over.

The first time I purely listen.

The second time I take notes.

Subsequent times I just keep listening, gleaning new bits of information each time.

At the end of the twelve weeks I have lost eight kilograms, exactly the amount I had gained.

I am totally stoked and eagerly enroll in the next round.

To say I am disappointed in round two of 12WBT would be an understatement.

I realise Michelle Bridges is a busy woman, and I don't expect it to be all new, but I also didn't expect it to be exactly the same.

Exactly. The. Same.

The 'newness' of the program is gone.

The 1200 calories per day seems too restrictive.

The mindset component is repetitive.

When I go to the forums looking for support I get harpooned by Michelle-supporters who won't allow anyone to voice anything other than how awesome Michelle is.

Jeeze I wasn't having a whine. I was just trying to give voice to my struggles.

I feel alone.

I bomb out of round two of 12WBT.

I gain five kilograms by the end of it.

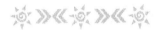

My period is late.

My period is never late.

I pick up a three-pack of pregnancy tests from the supermarket on the way home from work. I read the directions and decide to test immediately, even though it says morning urine is best.

The test is negative.

The following morning I test again. Still negative.

I wait four incredibly long days and test again, still negative.

My period is over a week late. This has never happened before, I am usually as regular as clockwork.

When Jeremy and I got married we were unsure of whether to have children and so we decided to put off making the call until I turned twenty eight.

Well I am twenty eight now; maybe this is the time.

I madly start googling false-negative pregnancy statistics.

Perhaps I really am pregnant.

Maybe the packet of tests were out of date.

I decide to tell Jeremy what is going on. We sit down and have our first real discussion about having children that we have had in ten years.

We decide it's time.

I am a bit excited about the possibility of being pregnant.

My period starts.

Well there goes that idea.

I am 92 kilograms and not pregnant, just fat.

Back to google for the answer to my weight problem.

I scroll the internet for hours, looking up all kinds of weight loss programs.

I stumble across a weight loss retreat on the sunshine coast. It's less than two hours away.

I see the contact number, my cursor is hovering as I debate what to do.

What have I got to lose?

Ummm it's fat camp, how about your dignity?

Your ass?

It's only 25 kilograms you don't need this

Do you want to get to over 100 kilograms again you fat fuck?

I pick up the phone and dial.

"Hello Meg speaking," answers a friendly voice.

"Erm Hi, mynameisSuzanneandI'mcallingaboutthe-fatcamp," I spit out before taking a huge breath.

"I am so sorry love, I think we have a bad line, can you say that again?" she replies.

I immediately like this Meg, trying to hide my faux paus with politeness. I feel she might be 'the one' to finally get me.

"This is Suzanne. I am calling for information about your weight loss retreat," I say.

"Suzanne, lovely to speak with you. My retreat is actually booked out until the new year. But, this is the most fortunate of timing, as I have literally just had a cancellation for the last week of next month's retreat. Are you interested?"

She then proceeds to give me all the details of what is involved. It sounds like exactly what I need. But there are no prices on the website so I am a bit nervous about how much this is going to cost. When I finally get the nerve to ask she replies, "only $1800".

Only $1800? For a week? WOW fat camp is a lot more expensive than I realised.

What the heck, that's what credit cards are for right?

I give her my details, and it's a done deal.

With fat camp booked in I feel so much better about my weight. This is going to be 'The Thing.'

Jeremy and I have a discussion about children and decide after the non-pregnancy we are ready to start trying for a baby.

The time leading up to fat camp flies by. When it's time to go I am feeling really nervous.

I check and triple check I have everything packed. I even buy tampons because my period is due while on camp and I don't want to miss out on the swimming because camp is at the beach. I hate tampons, but I hate being fat more.

I really need to stop calling this fat camp I think to myself on the drive down. *What if I accidentally call it that in front of the other participants?*

When I arrive at the fat camp, erm retreat, I fall immediately in love with the location. The resort is right by the beach, it is set up with villas spread around a lagoon with a giant inflatable in the middle that you can jump on. There are swimming pools in various locations, and bike riding tracks.

Pure bliss.

I scan the numbers of the villas, looking for number 331. I find it and hesitantly knock.

The door is flung open and before I can prepare myself a fit, tanned, pocket rocket of a woman flies out and embraces me in a giant hug.

"You must be Suzanne. I'm Meg. We have been waiting for you."

I momentarily forgot that fat camp had been going for the previous two weeks so most of the participants already knew each other. It was just me arriving for the last week on the cancellation deal.

"Come in. Come and meet everyone," says Meg, practically dragging me through the door.

Is this lady for real? Is she seriously this bubbly or is it all an act?

Before I can ponder this any further I am faced with the other 'campers'. Meg quickly does a round of introductions.

"Everyone this is Suzanne. Suzanne this is Shane, Brian, Margaret and Heather. Heather will be your roommate."

Shane is by far the largest. Both in stature and weight. I would guess he would be around 200 kilograms. He is sitting on the couch in sweat-stained grey shorts and a too small black singlet. He glares at me.

Brian has the most curly black hair I have ever seen, it's almost in ringlets and he gives me a friendly smile. I estimate him to be about thirty kilograms overweight.

Heather has long hair, and it's so straight I wonder if it's naturally that way or if she spends time straightening it every morning. She is around the same height and weight as me.

Margaret is thin. Like rail thin. Incredibly pale with saggy sallow skin. Her hair hangs listlessly around her like it's just given up on life. *Why on Earth is she even here?* I wonder for a moment if I am in the right place.

Before I can run for the door Heather sidles up to me and whispers,

"Don't mind Margaret, none of the rest of us know why she is here either."

I am momentarily stunned. *Were my thoughts that obvious?*

Heather smiles. "Come with me and I will show you our room."

The villa is grand and spacious. There are three floors. The top floor is the 'penthouse' which is where Shane's room is. The middle floor that we were currently on had the kitchen, living area, Brian's room and patio.

The ground floor had Margaret's room, the laundry, a bathroom, toilet, and finally Heather and my room. The boys both had ensuites so I was relieved it would be an all girl bathroom.

"I am so glad that you are here," Heather said. "Shane is a stick in the mud who sneaks out and buys treats. Margaret rarely leaves her room. Brian is ok. Barb, who was here before you came, cried all the time and was always on the phone to her kids moaning about how much she missed them. Meg has told us that you've already lost fifty kilograms! So I have been dying to meet you."

Before I can respond Meg appears in the doorway.

"Time to work out ladies," she says joyfully. "We need to burn at least one thousand calories before lunch."

I grab my heart rate monitor.

"Let's do this," I say.

Fat camp runs pretty much like I thought it would.

6am meet downstairs for green juice

6:15am walk to beach for first workout of the day

8am breakfast protein smoothie and shower

9am group theory session

11am work out at gym

1pm lunch

2pm group theory session

3pm free time - optional extra workout out

4pm pool session

5pm free time

6pm dinner

7:30pm bed because I am so exhausted from the big day

I struggle with the protein smoothie every morning. Each time I go to drink it I have flashbacks to my Tony Ferguson days and literally gag.

But if I don't drink it then it's a LONG time until lunch.

There are no snacks allowed.

I struggle without snacks.

I am tempted to ask Shane to smuggle me back some snacks on his 'walks' where we all know he is really heading up to the main reception vending machines. But Shane glares at me every time he sees me, so I would rather starve then ask him a favour.

On the fourth day a guest instructor arrives to take us through a yoga session instead of our usual morning gym session.

THE BEGINNING IS SH*T

I have never really been one for yoga. It's slow and boring, and I can't stand lying still at the end for savasana. I tend to fall asleep and constantly worry that I will snore.

It's a beautiful morning, and I am enjoying soaking up the sun when the guest instructor arrives.

"Namaste, my name is Carol, it's lovely to meet you," she reaches out to embrace me.

Holy cow this lady smells amazing. Whatever she is wearing I need some.

"What perfume are you wearing?" I ask

"Pardon?" she says

"Your perfume, it's awesome, what is it please?" I say

She chuckles. "I didn't put any on this morning. But yesterday I wore Jasmine."

We start the class, and I really enjoy it. Perhaps my views of yoga are changing. Or perhaps I really needed a break from the gym sessions.

On the sixth day of fat camp it is hot.

Really stinking hot.

I cannot wait for the afternoon pool session. As we walk back from the gym I am tempted to launch into the pool fully clothed. I am absolutely dripping with sweat.

My period is once again late, which normally would bother me, but after last month I figure there is something wrong with my cycle.

I am grateful for the reprieve and enjoy my time in the pool.

The seventh and final day of fat camp arrives, and before breakfast we are to weigh in. I started the camp at 92 kilograms, and I am really hoping that I have made it under the 90 kilo mark. It's been many months since I have lost two kilograms in a week.

I nervously step on the scales.

I am too scared to look down, but I hear Meg's sharp intake of breath as she records the number.

Shit, have I gained? Just my luck that I would be the first person in fat camp history to gain weight. Oh well at least I will get my money back.

The money back guarantee had been the cincher when it came to making up my mind to attend.

"You've lost five kilograms Suzanne. That is the biggest loss for a female we have ever had. Congratulations love, you deserve this."

Five kilograms? F-I-V-E.

I am absolutely stoked. I want to jump up and down. Ring my Mum. Scream from the rooftops all at once.

I walk out of the retreat feeling every one of those five kilograms lighter and I head home.

The next morning I am super keen for some real breakfast. If I never touch another bloody green juice or protein smoothie as long as I live I will be a happy woman.

I eagerly open the pantry and grab out my weetbix and just looking at the box I feel a roll of nausea. Oh no. No, no no.

I can't be pregnant!

Of course you can be pregnant you dumbass! What have you been trying for the last month for?

I put the weetbix box back and grab the car keys, and head off to the supermarket to get a pregnancy test.

I sit the pregnancy test on the bench and look at it all day long. I don't want to do the test on my own. I wait for Jeremy to get back from work.

As soon as he walks in I brandish the test at him.

"Let's do this," I say, marching resolutely to the bathroom.

He waits patiently for me to take the test, and I bring it out and we sit it on the table.

"How long do we have to wait?" he asks.

"Three minutes."

When three minutes are up, there is the tiniest of faint lines in the second box.

Jeremy is so excited he jumps up and throws his hands in the air shouting, "We're pregnant!"

I watch him being so excited, and I have tunnel vision. The sides of the room are literally starting to cave in, and I can't quite digest this information.

I feel like one of those cartoon characters who have been hit on the head and you see the birds start to cycle around their head.

I'm having a baby. I will literally have to look after another person for the rest of my life. I won't be able to go to the gym anymore because I will be a mother. I am going to gain all the weight back. I am going to have to lose it all over again. I don't know if I can do this anymore.

The thoughts are whirling so fast that I feel dizzy.

Chapter Nine

I sit in the waiting room at the doctors surgery fidgeting in my chair.

I am nervous about the pregnancy, and we haven't told anyone yet so I am bursting to share the news.

As I shuffle around in the chair I enjoy the feeling of spaciousness, the sides don't dig into my bottom, and I feel a sense of freedom.

I worry about gaining weight with this pregnancy. The constant worry about regaining all of my lost weight is really sucking the joy out of what should be a happy time.

You shouldn't feel like this, you should be lucky that you even got pregnant. Some people struggle.

If you lose this baby it will serve you right for being so selfish. You shouldn't be focusing on you right now, it's about what's best for the baby.

I feel really isolated. I don't have anyone to share these thoughts with. I am debating how to raise my concerns.

"Suzanne," I hear my name called, and I am snapped out of dark thoughts.

Before Dr Ashley has even closed the door, I shout, "I'm pregnant!"

"Well I don't handle pregnancy, so I will need to refer you to a colleague". He replies.

I have been waiting two weeks to tell someone, and this is the response I get? What a let-down.

"Book in to see Dr Gough when you're about 10 weeks along" he says.

"I have so many questions now. What about my exercise? Wha-"

He cuts me off. "You don't want to put any stress on the baby by raising your heart rate too high, so just walking and swimming and keep your heart rate below 140 at all times."

"Bu-" I try again.

"As I told you Suzanne, I am not a baby doctor. You can ask Dr Gough the rest of your questions when you see him."

I am concerned about what I might have done to my baby at the retreat. I had often pushed myself to a maximum heart rate of 180-190.

Have I cooked my poor baby's brain?

I had been planning to go to the gym on my way home from the doctor's. I couldn't go now. I go straight home.

I'm restless. I can't stop thinking about the damage I might have done to bub. Before I know it I find myself in the kitchen, mindlessly opening and closing the fridge.

Can't eat. Don't want to get fat.

Can't exercise. Don't want to cook my baby.
Can't tell anyone. I am not twelve weeks along yet.
I am driving myself crazy.

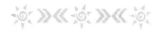

The day of my twelve week scan finally arrives. I am super excited to finally be able to see bub. Jeremy isn't able to come because he has some big meeting at work. I am scared to go alone, so I invite Laura to come with me.

I don't know which one of us is more excited.

After drinking what feels like more water than humanly possible I wait uncomfortably to be called in.

"I need to pee," I complain to Laura.

"It won't be much longer," she reassures me.

"I seriously am going to wet myself." I say with some urgency.

"If you do that you will have to start this process all over again," she reminds me gently.

Dammit why does she have to be so logical?

"My appointment was supposed to be over an hour ago," I complain. "Surely being pregnant is torture enough."

Am I this much of a whiny bitch normally?

Surely it's the pregnancy hormones.

"Suzanne," a male voice calls from the doorway.

As soon as I stand I am really worried about how I will make it across the room. My appointment was scheduled for over an hour ago, and being the over achiever that I am, I had drunk an extra litre of water for good measure. I literally feel like I am about to burst.

I shuffle like a geisha across the room to the voice from the doorway and hot damn he is gorgeous. Six foot tall, tanned, blond hair, blue eyes; he looks more like he belongs at the beach than at an ultrasound joint. I nudge Laura in the ribs and widen my eyes.

"Could you be any more obvious?" she hisses at me.

I giggle and then am immediately reminded of my bladder situation. Damn it.

I lie down on the table and Adonis smears the cold goop on my belly.

"Are you ready to see bub?" he says.

"Yessssssssss"

"Well I am sorry Suzanne but your bladder is too full," he says

"Ummm excuse me?" I say.

"You're going to have to go and let a little bit out," he tells me.

"Let a little bit out?" I screech "how am I supposed to do that?"

I shuffle off to the bathroom.

Letting a little bit out is every bit as awkward and uncomfortable as I had imagined it would be. I get the job done, eager to see bub.

When I return, we try again and sure enough bub is jumping around like a jelly bean. I get all the images put on CD, and am super keen to show Jeremy when he gets home from work.

Jeremy calls me in the afternoon. I assume he wants to know how the ultrasound went and I am keen to tell him. Before I can get a word in he says, "Suze, I just got made redundant."

What. The. Fuck?

I had given up work a few months ago. I was planning to be a stay at home Mum. Jeremy's work was the primary employer for the town. There was no way he was going to find another job anywhere in the region. We were going to have to move.

Well shit.

"What's your job title again?" I ask him.

Ever the 'Miss fix it', or perhaps it's the pregnancy hormones. Either way, I take charge and go straight to google.

Before Jeremy even makes it home, I have shortlisted a half dozen jobs he can apply for. Located his CV ready for him to brush up.

He submits his applications that night.

The next day he got a call from a job in the Hunter Valley in New South Wales.

The following week they fly him down for a face to face interview.

They offer him the job that same afternoon.

Within a week we had gone from redundant, oh fuck, to brand new job.

Pity about having to move interstate, but shit happens.

We pack up our house. Farewell Kingaroy early on a Saturday morning. Jump in the car and start driving.

The drive takes a lot longer than anticipated, thanks to the pregnancy hormones meaning I have to pee every few kilometers. We overnight it in Tamworth and arrive in Singleton on Sunday.

Jeremy starts his new job on the Monday.

I am nothing short of an action taker.

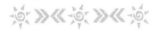

The pregnancy is hard, I am nauseous day in and day out, it doesn't let up like I hoped it would.

I suffer from migraines regularly, and often spend entire days in bed hoping they will pass.

Prior to pregnancy I had been very active, and now I only walk and go to water aerobics twice per week.

The interstate move is hard. It took me years to get established in Kingaroy, and find friends, and now I am once again alone.

I reach out on facebook and connect with some other expecting mothers in town. It's good to start to build a social network.

I gain a lot of weight in pregnancy. I average a kilogram per week.

At my 38 week check up, my GP notices my blood pressure is elevated, and I have trace proteins in my urine, so he decides it's best to refer me to Maitland hospital to take over my care.

I had been planning to deliver at Singleton hospital, which is five minutes from home. Maitland is over forty minutes away.

Because of my blood pressure and proteins they are concerned about preeclampsia, and so I have to be monitored daily. In Maitland. Each time I visit I see a different doctor, and the plan moving forward changes.

I dread driving in each day, not sure what the doctor of the day is going to decide.

I am sent for an ultrasound, and it's declared that my baby is going to be at least eleven pounds.

Great, I am carrying King Kong.

At the following visit the latest doctor decides to induce me on my due date.

I have mixed feelings about this. I would hate to go through labour only to end up with a c-section.

I mention my concerns and ask about an elective c-section. I'm told we will do an 8 hour trial of labour, and if that fails we can move to a c-section.

8 hours doesn't seem too bad. I'm not exactly ecstatic, but I consent to this approach.

I arrive at the hospital on my due date with my suitcase and proceed to the desk to fill in the required paperwork.

"Why are you being induced?" asks the nurse at the desk.

"Because my baby is predicted to be at least eleven pounds," I reply.

"We don't induce based on size prediction. Go home and we will sort this out tomorrow," she says.

I turn to waddle away.

"Oh, before you go we better check your vitals and urine" she says.

Due to my growing belly it's getting harder and harder to pee in the cup, good thing I am flexible.

The nurse takes my blood pressure and frowns. I am used to this response so I am not concerned. She then dips the stick in my urine and declares, "Well you are not going home until you have this baby Missy."

Wow she changed her tune fast.

"Your blood pressure is very high and you have three plus proteins in your urine, so it's time we bring this baby out, okay?"

Honestly, I am a little annoyed. *First she wants me to go home, now she wants me to stay.*

She explains to me how the cervidil tape works, they will insert it, I will be admitted for observation because of my blood pressure and protein in my urine. In the morning the tape will be removed and all going well they will break my waters. If I am not dilated enough they will insert a balloon.

The insertion of the cervidil isn't comfortable, but I have had worse. I am admitted to my room and then left on my own.

Jeremy is at work. He doesn't have much annual leave accrued having only just started the job, and I don't want him to waste it until the baby is actually coming. So I call him and give him an update of what is happening. I tell him I will phone him if labour starts.

The following morning at 6am the cervidil is removed. I am told I am dilated enough, but there are no birthing suites available, so I am sent back to my room to wait until they have a space.

I wait.

I walk up and down the hallway as I have heard that walking can bring on labour. No luck.

I go outside and walk with one foot on the curb and one on the ground because I hear that can induce labour. Nothing.

I wander across the road to the pub and order a spicy curry for lunch. Still nothing.

I have to keep returning to my room every hour so that my blood pressure can be monitored. Some nurses whisper about a c-section. But the doctor on shift is adamant about a 'trial of labour.'

When I ask what that means, she tells me that they will give me eight hours of labour and if no baby, then I will be sent for a c-section.

At 5pm there is finally a birthing suite free. I phone Jeremy and tell him to come in now; it's finally time.

Jeremy comes flying in at 5:30pm, even though it's a forty minute drive.

It's a bit of a hurry up and wait scenario as we wait for a doctor to break my waters. At 6pm she finally arrives. She does the check and tells me that though I am dilated enough, she doesn't want to break my waters because bub is not engaged, and there is a risk of cord prolapse if they do it now.

So it's time for the balloon.

The insertion of the balloon is tortuous. Just when I think it can't get any more excruciating, they inflate it. I feel like I have to wee.

Immediately. I cry, I whinge, I complain.

"This is normal," the nurse reassures me "The balloon is dilating your cervix further. You will get used to the pressure."

"Pressure?" I say. "This isn't bloody pressure! It hurts like hell, and I want it out. I want this *baby* out. I am just done. Can I have a c-section and just be over with this?"

"You have to have your trial of labour," she tells me. "It will all be over soon. Go back to your room, and we will remove the balloon in the morning."

Jeremy leads me back to my room. He then tells me he will be back in the morning. I barely hear him. I head straight to the toilet. I swear I am going to wee myself. I sit down and nothing comes out; it's just the pressure of the balloon.

It is the longest night of my life. I literally go back and forth to the toilet on repeat. I get no sleep. The pain is intense. But no contractions.

At 5am the following morning I am led once more to the birthing suite.

"You are going to meet your baby today." A happy registrar exclaims.

Really? Is today really going to be the day? I have been here since Wednesday, it's now Saturday, and I just want to go home.

The balloon is removed.

My waters are broken.

The drip is inserted.

At 7am my contractions finally start.

12pm I can't take the pain anymore, and I ask for some gas.

12:05pm I have a reaction to the gas and start vomiting everywhere.

My blood pressure is taken, and it's 180/110.

"Suzanne you need an epi-dural." I am told.

"No epi-dural!"

"Suzanne we need to bring your blood pressure down now. You need an epi-dural."

We argue back and forth for what feels like forever and eventually I concede. I sign the paperwork.

6pm the epidural is inserted.

Absolute bliss. I can't feel a thing.

My contractions start to slow down. So they administer another drug. The vomiting comes back worse than before. They give me something else to stop the vomiting. I am so relieved.

Then I feel like something is crawling under my skin. I start shrieking and ripping at my arms.

They give me something else. My head begins to ache. Like I have been hit on one side of the face with an axe. The throbbing is nearly unbearable.

11pm - I am fully dilated, it's finally time to push. The nurses call up to theatre, "You can all go home," she tells the team on standby. "She's fully dilated, and we are about to meet this baby."

Two hours later, still no baby.

Suddenly my contractions just stop.

"Suzanne you need a c-section," the midwife says.

"No fucking way. I can do this."

"Honey, you are no longer contracting," she says gently.

"Pump me full of more drugs. I can do this."

"Suzanne you have maxed out your Syntocinon. We can't give you anymore. You need a c-section," she replies.

While she is explaining this to me, the other midwife is calling the theatre to arrange for a team and my transport.

"Lady, I wanted a fucking C-section days ago, but instead I did what I was told. I've been poked, prodded, shoved and stabbed. I am NOT going to be cut too. Let's get this fucking thing out!" I snap.

"Let me get the doctor." she says.

The same registrar that broke my waters and told me I was going to meet my baby today, walks in.

"Have you been home?" I growl.

"Pardon me?"

"Have you been working since I saw you yesterday, or have you been home?"

I am not going to be cut open by someone who has been on her feet the entire time I have been in labour!

"Oh honey, I broke your waters and went home. But I am fresh as a daisy now. Let's get this baby out. Today is the day you are going to meet your baby" she says happily.

I've heard that one before.

"I think I must be carrying Renesmee" I say.

"Pardon?" she says.

Obviously not a Twilight fan.

They wheel me into the theatre alone.

Eventually Jeremy is allowed to join me. He looks funny in scrubs.

After what feels like a lifetime, at 3:16am, on Sunday the 30th of June, five days after my induction started, Xanthe is finally delivered.

Chapter Ten

The next morning I transfer back to Singleton Hospital. I never want to set foot in Maitland Hospital again.

I may not have got the birth I wanted, but come hell or highwater, I am going to breastfeed. Xanthe is a great latcher, apparently this is a good thing. But when she feeds she sucks so hard I feel like my eyeballs are going to be dragged backward out of my head and then down out through my boobs.

She never stops feeding.

The nurse gives me a log book to fill in whenever I feed. I diligently fill in the details, for the entire day and hand it to her the next morning when she comes back on shift.

She scans the paper.

"Suzanne, darling, you're only supposed to record the times that she feeds."

"I have been."

"But, honey, according to this she has pretty much been at your breast for twenty of the last twenty-four hours. That can't be right," She says.

"She has been."

"Oh no, darling, you're just tired. Fill it in properly today, and I will review it again tomorrow. Remember, just record the times she is actually on the breast."

She walks out of the room.

Xanthe doesn't sleep at all.

When she isn't at my breast trying to suck out my eyeballs, she is screaming the ward down.

That night an angel appears — well it is a new midwife, but to me she is an angel — and offers to take her so that I can get some sleep.

Xanthe hasn't had any dirty, or even wet, nappies. She still has the crystals. So they decide to weigh her, she has gone from 4.2 kilograms at birth to 3.5 kilograms. So I am sent home from the hospital with a referral to see a lactation consultant.

I do everything the lactation consultant suggests.

I put Xanthe to each breast for thirty minutes to feed. Then I pump each breast for fifteen minutes. This whole process takes one and a half hours, and I have to do it every two hours.

I have thirty minutes to myself to eat, drink and pee and the process starts all over again.

Xanthe still hasn't had a dirty or wet nappy, she just has some orange dust in her nappy when we change her. She is still losing weight.

"We are going to have to start topping her up with formula," says the lactation consultant. "After each feed you can give her 20ml of formula. Only 20ml. This is just a stop gap until your supply increases."

I cry as I walk into the pharmacy to buy the formula.

I feel like such a failure. I couldn't deliver my baby, and now I can't feed her.

Is it because I am fat?

Did my weight do this?

I gained over forty kilograms in my pregnancy, did that somehow stunt my ability to be a mother?

I bring all the items home from the pharmacy, and I stand at the sink and cry.

I don't know how to do this.

I never researched formula as the birthing classes told me breast is best.

How do I even use this steriliser?

I try to read the tiny writing on the instructions, but I can't see through my tears.

Xanthe screams even louder.

Jeremy had to go straight back to work the day after Xanthe was born because he had no annual leave saved, and being in a new job he has no paternity leave entitlements.

I figure out the formula and Xanthe drinks the 20mls in no time at all. For a blessed few moments she is blissfully quiet. It isn't long before the screaming starts again.

The following day I go visit the child health nurse, Rebecca.

"How are you going Suzanne?" she asks kindly.

"I'm fine," I lie.

"You can tell me whatever you need to love. This is a safe space," she prompts.

At this moment Xanthe begins to wail. Loudly.

"It's ok, Suzanne, I have all the time in the world, you can feed her."

I go through the process of feeding Xanthe both sides, and then I fumble for the formula. I give her the 20ml. She continues to wail.

"Would you like to give her a bit more?" Rebecca asks.

"Oh no, I can't give her more," I say.

"Why not?"

"Because the lactation consultant said 20mls and no more."

Rebecca points at a poster on the wall, one of many posters that are around the room of newborn babies sleeping peacefully.

"Suzanne, has your baby ever looked like this?" she asks kindly.

I look at the floor. I look out the window. I begin to shake. I quickly put Xanthe down, less I drop her.

Keep it together. Keep it together. Keep it together.

I can't keep it together any longer.

"No. She has never looked like that at all," I say in a small voice.

"What would be the harm in giving her just a little bit more formula? Just enough so that she can have a good sleep. You can have a good sleep too. You will feel like a new woman."

"I...I couldn't do that. I need to get my milk to come in."

"Some women can't breastfeed, Suzanne, and there is no shame in that."

"Less than 1% of women," I say. "The rest just don't try hard enough."

"Suzanne, you have tried so hard. You have fed, pumped, you've taken all the supplements. You have baked the lactation cookies. You have taken prescription medication that you've told me is making you feel un- well. There is nothing more you could do. Now you need to take care of yourself."

"I am taking care of myself. Everything is fine."

"Honey, your shirt is inside out and backwards."

I burst out laughing, I can't help it. The laughing quickly turns into crying. Shoulder shaking sobbing.

Rebecca reaches over and gives me a hug.

"You're an amazing Mum. Xanthe is lucky to have you. A little bit of extra formula for a happy baby. A happy baby makes a happy Mum. It's a win:win."

I reflect on what she said and for the rest of the day I give Xanthe an extra 20ml formula. Then an extra 40ml of formula. She sleeps for four straight hours that night.

Rebecca was right. I do feel like a new woman.

The following day at our visit, I excitedly update the lactation consultant. Her response is less than ideal.

"60ml! You gave her 60ml at her feed. Why did you do that? I specifically told you no more than 20ml!" She exclaims.

I immediately feel deflated. The buoyed feeling from the sleep is forgotten.

She continues to lecture me about my milk coming in and how formula will make Xanthe a lazy feeder.

I try to tell her it's been so long that I really don't think my milk is going to come in now, but she won't hear of it.

At the end of the appointment I ask her when she'd like me to come back in.

"I am busy over the next few days. I will call you to arrange a time," she says dismissively.

This is the first time this has happened. Every other time we have made the appointment at the end of the session, and it's never been more than three days between visits.

I don't hear from her again.

I feel abandoned.

I continue to take Xanthe weekly to see the child health nurse, Rebecca. When she is six weeks old Xanthe has finally reached her birth weight again.

I persist with mix feeding until she is three months old. By that time she is drinking upwards of 120ml of formula per feed and so I decide to quit breast feeding.

I read online all these horror stories about stopping breastfeeding suddenly.

I read about mastitis and other such things. I don't know if this will be an issue for me because I don't understand what it feels like to have full breasts. I never noticed any changes throughout my pregnancy or post birth. Funnily enough my breasts were the only part of me that didn't change size, despite the forty kilogram weight gain.

My worries were unfounded. I stop feeding and nothing happens. Well, except for gaining many hours back in my day.

Rebecca refers me to see a social worker.

I am resistant to go at first, but she encourages me and reluctantly I attend.

The social worker diagnoses me with PTSD. I feel like even more of a failure.

What kind of weak person gets PTSD from childbirth? Isn't that for people who go to war and get shot at? Or police who see all sorts of violent crime?

I resist this diagnosis. I love seeing the social worker, though, because she makes me feel like I am not alone, and I can be truly honest.

Among all my mum friends with their breastfeeding and their sleeping babies and their bliss, I feel like a total outsider and failure.

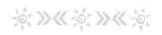

Eventually we settle into a routine. Xanthe is never fond of being put down, she much prefers to be carried. She hates the car, the pram, the floor. The only time she seems to be calm is when she is held.

I invest in an ergo baby carrier. But I am far too fat to do it up properly. Fortunately you can purchase an extender for the waist strap.

Although Xanthe loves it, I can't stand it. It's big and bulky and makes it difficult to do things. Not to mention carrying her on the front puts a big strain on my back.

I try in vain to lose weight.

Firstly I try the traditional method of Weight Watchers. I feel almost like I am doing the walk of shame going back to meetings again. I manage to drop 9 kilograms before throwing in the towel.

It took me six weeks to lose those nine kilograms and only three weeks to regain it all.

I join 12WBT again. Not even committing to a full week before quitting.

I flit about from diet to diet but I don't really commit to anything.

I decide to try crossfit.

I love it.

It's high intensity. The music is loud, and the people are crazy fit. But I am not made to feel out of place. Even though I am literally twice the size of the other women.

I jump into their 12-week challenge.

At week 4 I hurt my back. Once again I am laid up in bed.

It takes me a month to recover.

By the time I am ready to go again the crossfit box has closed.

I don't have the stamina to commit to something else, and so I just quit.

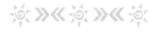

When Xanthe is nine months old I return to work.

I go back to Medicare, but this time I take a job in a call centre. It takes me over an hour to drive into work each day, and obviously the same distance home. That is nearly two and a half hours in the car each day.

Being in a call centre I work a desk job. So that is another eight hours of sitting down.

I gain weight faster than ever before.

Xanthe doesn't sleep through the night. She often wakes three to four times. Coupled with the driving and the work, I feel pretty much like a zombie.

I eat a lot of take away. Often grabbing Maccas for dinner on the way home. Sometimes I mix it up and have Hungry Jacks instead.

Although initially I had wanted two children close together, I can't even entertain the thought of another child.

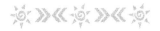

When Xanthe is fifteen months old, Jeremy is made re-dundant yet again.

Effective immediately.

I increase my work hours to full time, we remove Xanthe from daycare, and Jeremy stays home to look after her.

A week after finding out Jeremy has no job I realise my period is late.

My period is never late.

I dismiss it as being due to stress. Jeremy has just lost his job. I have increased my work hours to full time. I think nothing of it.

It's not possible to be pregnant at this size, right? People who weigh well over 100kg struggle to conceive.

After a week when my period has still not arrived, I call into the supermarket on the way home and buy a test.

The traffic is heavy, and I don't get home till after 9pm.

I am exhausted, but want to know straight away if we're pregnant or not. So I pee on the stick.

"I'm grabbing a shower," I say to Jeremy "Can you check this test after three minutes. I'm sure it's negative, but I just did it for peace of mind."

No sooner have I turned on the water and stepped in the shower when Jeremy follows me into the bathroom.

"There's two lines, so that's negative right?" He says.

"WHAT?!" I screech, flying out of the shower and snatching it off him.

"This can't be right" I say.

I violently shake the test. As if somehow that will shake the second line away.

"Shit, shit, shit!"

"It's going to be okay," Jeremy reassures.

"How is this going to be okay? I am our only source of income, and I am pregnant. Do you remember last time I was pregnant? I was nauseous everyday and I suffered from frequent migraines. What are we going to do?"

"We will figure it out," he says.

The following morning I take another pregnancy test in hopes that the first one was wrong.

It wasn't.

Still pregnant.

With great trepidation, I tentatively step on the bathroom scale. Lifting each foot and lowering it gently, as if that will somehow make the number smaller.

145kg.

Fuck.

Chapter Eleven

I make an appointment with the same GP I saw for my pregnancy with Xanthe. By my estimate I am about six weeks along. The very first thing he does is weigh me.

"Suzanne you are 145 kilograms. Your BMI is too high to deliver at Singleton Hospital. Your pregnancy is moderate risk."

"I won't go to Maitland," I say.

"Well you can deliver at John Hunter in Newcastle."

"Done."

"Whatever you do, don't gain any weight this pregnancy," He warns.

How helpful.

Does any doctor ever congratulate you on being pregnant in real life? Or is that just something that happens on TV?

I really want to have this baby in a private hospital. We have private health insurance. But we can't afford the excess, as I am the only one working.

When I am fifteen weeks along Jeremy lands a six month contract in Brisbane.

We decide not to move to Brisbane as a family. His job offer is not ongoing. We have bought a house in the

Hunter Valley. I have a job. So he will fly to Brisbane to work, and come home every second weekend.

When I am eighteen weeks pregnant I put Xanthe down for her lunch time nap and go to make myself a cup of tea. I hear Xanthe crying, it gets louder and she sounds distressed.

I open the door to her room and I see her in the corner of the cot that is pushed against the wall.

She doesn't move towards me as I go into the room like she normally would.

Instead her crying just gets louder and louder.

I feel dread pooling in the pit of my stomach as I realise she has tried to climb out of the cot and has gotten her leg stuck between bars.

I don't know what to do.

I begin to panic.

Should I call the fire brigade?

How long will it take the fire brigade to get here?

Does she have any blood supply to that leg?

While the thoughts are racing through my mind I realise the very first thing I need to do is get to her.

I can't reach her as she's jammed up in the corner. So I grab the sides and lift the cot out away from the wall.

The cot is heavy wood, and the second I lift it I feel a tearing sensation across my abdomen. I ignore the pain while I finally reach Xanthe.

Her leg is stuck and stuck good. It's bright red and swollen and she is screaming so loud I can't even think.

I run to the garage and get a saw and run back to the cot.

This will take too long to cut.

Breathe, just breathe.

I go to the fridge, and I get some butter, and I lather her leg with it. Slowly and methodically, I manage to squeeze it back between the bars.

Later that afternoon I go to a friend's place for a play date.

My stomach is really hurting from lifting the cot. I am unsure what to do. I relay the story to my friends. They look at each other worriedly.

"I will look after Xanthe, and Denise will take you to the hospital. Just get a check up and see that everything is good with bub," says Bella calmly.

Singleton hospital isn't far away. The trip doesn't even take us ten minutes.

I explain what happened to the triage nurse, and I am taken straight into the emergency department. By this time it's around 5pm in the afternoon.

A midwife approaches with doppler in hand.

"Let's check on this bub," she says with a smile.

She spends a few minutes running the doppler over my belly.

"You're how far along?" She asks.

"18 weeks."

"Have you heard bub's heart on doppler yet?" she asks.

"Yes, last week at my GP."

"Ok, cool. Well this machine has always been a bit dodgy. Let me go grab the other one."

She returns a few minutes later with a second machine and a second nurse.

They spend what feels like forever searching for the heartbeat. They look at each other and then back at me.

"Well, Suzanne, we can't find the heartbeat. But that may be because you are…well because of….well due to your size." She finally gets the words out.

"I am sure there is nothing to worry about. Just make an appointment with your GP in the morning, and get him to check you out. If needed, he can refer you for an ultrasound. We would do it, but we don't have an ultrasound machine here. If you get any pain or bleeding before then, please go to Maitland hospital."

Denise drives me back to Bella's place to get Xanthe. I reassure them both that I am totally fine. I take Xanthe home and put her to bed. Then I pace.

Is bub ok? Is it really just that I am too fat to find a pulse?

What the fuck was I thinking lifting that cot?

No way in hell am I going to Maitland for an ultrasound! Should I drive myself to Newcastle and get checked out now?

Eventually I go to bed, but I don't sleep. I lie awake worrying. It's almost a relief when Xanthe wakes up at 4am. It's something to distract me until the doctor's surgery opens.

I phone the surgery right at 8:30. Before the receptionist has even finished her spiel, I interrupt her and almost shout, "It's Suzanne Culberg, I need to see Dr Mitchell as soon as possible this morning please!"

"He doesn't have anything available today. I could possibly fit you in tomorrow afternoon, one moment while I check," she says.

"No, I need to see him right now. I was at..." before I can finish she cuts me off.

"I am sorry, but he is booked out for today. I will have a look..." she says

Feeling frustrated, I cut her off. "I was at Singleton hospital, they told me to see Dr Mitchell as soon as possible."

"Oh. Come straight away, and we will fit you in."

I am feeling even more flustered by this conversation. What was I thinking wasting time on the phone? I should have just gone straight in.

I drop Xanthe at daycare, and I go to the doctor's surgery. When I arrive the receptionist has a totally different manner than she did on the phone.

"Good morning, Suzanne. We just received a fax from the hospital. Dr Mitchell will see you next. In the meantime, come wait in the nurse's office." She smiles reassuringly.

Received a fax? Are we in 1986?

If there's nothing to worry about, why can't I wait in the regular waiting area like every other time?

Don't panic Suzanne. Just breathe.

As I sit in the nurse's office and stare at the wall, I am distracted by a sign that reads 'Keep Calm I'm a doctor.'

They're lucky I didn't start laughing hysterically.

It's not long before Dr Mitchell pokes his head around the corner and motions for me to follow him.

"I have your notes from the hospital, but in your own words what happened yesterday?" he asks kindly.

I fill him in on Xanthe being stuck, lifting the cot, and the pain and trip to the hospital.

"Have you experienced any further pain?" he asks.

"No. Nothing."

"Let's have a listen."

Without being asked, I hop up onto the table and pull up my shirt as he reaches for the gel and the doppler.

I hear the sound of the doppler; it's a scratchy kind of echo sound. My ears strain for the thump of a heart beat, but I hear nothing. Just the echo.

Dr Mitchell moves the doppler around. Still nothing. He keeps a very calm face and says to me, "Doppler can be unreliable, especially in someone of your size. Let's set up the portable ultrasound."

A few minutes later he is running the ultrasound over my belly. I can't see the screen, but I don't need to. I can see by the expression on his face that something is wrong.

I watch his forehead crinkle, his jaw tightening, his mouth moving around as he tries to select the right words.

"Suzanne," he says slowly, "I can see your baby, but I can't see a heartbeat."

I feel the blood rushing in my ears, and I don't want to hear the rest. I go to turn away but he looks me directly in the eyes and says, "There is no easy way to say this but it is likely that your baby is dead. We will need to send you for an official ultrasound to confirm."

I start crying. Shoulder-shaking sobs.

I did this.

If only I hadn't lifted that stupid cot.

What was I thinking?

This is all my fault.

"The nurse will help you get organised," he says. With that he calls the nurse. and she comes to collect me to take her back to her room. She sits me down and pats me on the shoulder.

"We will get you through this," she says.

She brings me a glass of water and a box of tissues and lets me know she is going to phone around to find me somewhere to do the ultrasound. I nod and listen to her begin making the calls.

While she is talking, I manage to bring my sobbing under control. I am now doing some weird kind of hiccup thing. I reach blindly for my phone debating whether to call Jeremy or my mum.

I decide to call no one. Not until I know for sure. No point worrying them further.

Deep down inside I have a small glimmer of hope.
Handheld ultrasounds are not the most accurate. I am
a very big woman. It's possible the baby is in a position
where the heartbeat can't be seen.

Dead. Dead. Dead.

Replaying the doctor's words in my head brings a
fresh wave of tears.

*They have to say it. You were taught this at medical
school. It's better not to give false hope.*

With all this internal dialogue going on I have lost
track of the nurse's phone calls. But once she has made the
appointment she comes back over to give me the details.

I reach for my bag.

"What are you doing?" she asks.

"Driving to Maitland for my ultrasound" I reply.

"Oh no no no, honey. I will call someone to drive you."

"It's fine. I can do it."

"No." She states firmly. "You are in no state to do
this. You have a young child at care, and you have to look
after yourself. Let me organise this all for you. Give me
your phone, tell me which friends I should call, and lie
back down while I sort it out."

I am so relieved I start crying all over again. She
brings me a fresh box of tissues.

Wow did I really go through a whole box already?

The nurse is amazing, she organises someone to pick
Xanthe up from care. Also, someone to get my car from
the doctor's surgery and drop it back to my place. Most

importantly she arranges for my friend Mel to pick me up and take me to my appointment. She also manages to chase up some sandwiches and a heat pack while I am waiting for Mel to arrive.

Mel arrives to take me to the appointment, also bearing food and a drink.

I am so grateful to both the nurse and Mel that it starts off another round of sobbing.

I don't think I have ever cried so much in my life.

Maitland is a forty minute drive, and the ultrasound lab is located at the private hospital which is renowned for its very limited parking.

"Don't worry," says Mel. "I always find a car park right out the front." She says in such an upbeat voice that I believe her.

She keeps the conversation going on the drive out there. Full credit to her, because I don't know if the roles had been reversed how I would have fared.

When we get there, sure enough a car is pulling out directly in front of the building. I marvel at our good luck.

"Would you like me to come in with you or wait in the car?" Mel asks.

"Come in please."

When we walk in, the place is crowded. It's full pandemonium with people everywhere.

"How about you let reception know that we are here, and I will find us some seats," Mel says.

I head over to the queue and wait my turn.

When I make it to the counter I shakingly hand over my medicare card and referral form.

The receptionist scans my details.

"Oh, Suzanne, yes I received a call about you. The cost of the scan is three hundred dollars, but if your baby is indeed deceased we will bulk bill you," she says.

With that I burst into tears all over again.

Loud, wailing tears.

I don't care who can see me. I don't care what I look like. All the calm I had managed to gather is instantly gone.

Mel appears by my side like an angel and musters me over to a chair. We don't have to wait long before my name is called. I am holding tight to Mel, as she helps me up from the chair and supports me into the room.

The sonographer tries to make some small talk but I am beyond being pleasant and I cut her short with, "I just want this fucking scan now. Let's get this over with."

I hold my breath as she smears on the gel and puts the wand to my belly.

I can't look at the screen.

"There's bub" she says moving the wand around, "and there's the heart beat, nice and strong."

I exhale.

"Are you sure?" I ask tentatively.

"Quite sure, have a look here at the screen," she says.

Mel is jumping up and down screaming.

The sonographer is smiling.

Slowly I turn my head towards the screen, and I see a little limb waving.

Intense relief surges throughout my body, and I feel like I can breathe again.

My baby is okay.

The confidence in her voice. The way she said it, it was like she had never had a doubt in the world.

I feel instantly guilty for swearing at her. I apologise profusely. She reassures me kindly that there are no worries at all, reminding me that I've had a big day.

My life has turned on a dime that day, in both directions.

Now all's right with the world again.

She does the full eighteen week scan. I had originally had it booked for the following week, but we decide to do it early because we are already there. Might as well make the most of it. There are a few images that she is unable to get clear shots of, so I make a follow up appointment for two weeks time.

Mel drops me home, and there is a gift waiting at the front door. While I was paying for the scan she had rung one of our other friends to get it organised. It's a bib, a bonnet and a plush rattle. The first items for this bub. I'm so appreciative.

Bella brings Xanthe back after daycare. Denise drops me off some dinner and offers to stay. I thank her profusely, but say I would rather be alone.

I am so grateful to have such amazing friends. It is wonderful how everyone has banded together and taken care of me.

The following day I call a private obstetrician. The receptionist tells me that I am too far into my pregnancy now, and he is fully booked. I burst into tears, and as I sob out my story, she tells me she will speak to him and get back to me.

She rings back an hour later and tells me he will take over my care, all I need is a referral from my GP.

I make the appointment, and I visit Dr Mitchell for the last time. I tell him that although I appreciate that it was a delicate situation, I just can't see him anymore. I ask for the referral for the private obstetrician, and I never go back there.

I find a whole different GP practice. From my very first appointment I know I have made the right choice. My new GP adores Xanthe and is most excited about my pregnancy. Also, she never once mentions my weight.

I am nervous about my appointment with the obstetrician. But he is absolutely amazing. He also never once mentions my weight, nor does he weigh me at any of my appointments. I am so relieved. It feels good to be able to relax in this pregnancy.

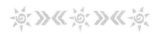

My pregnancy from here runs relatively smoothly. I have my heart set on a VBAC. Dr Smalls is completely supportive of this plan.

At 32 weeks my blood pressure starts to increase and so I am monitored more closely.

At 34 weeks the proteins appear in my urine again, and I am encouraged to rest where possible.

I finish up at work.

At 35 weeks I have a scan. Bub isn't in an ideal position for natural birth, and the baby has the cord around their neck. My blood pressure is steadily increasing, and Dr Smalls thinks it best to schedule a C-section.

Although disappointed, I agree.

At 36 weeks my blood pressure is bordering on concern, and Dr Smalls wants to admit me to hospital. I have no one to watch Xanthe. I ask a few of my friends, but no one is able. It's a big ask to take on an almost 2 year old. My family all live interstate, and Jeremy is still in Brisbane working his contract.

Dr Smalls agrees to let me stay home for now, but I have to have my blood pressure, urine and blood checked daily. If it goes past a certain level then he doesn't care what happens, I will have to go to hospital.

My dad flies up from Tasmania to help me take care of Xanthe, and to run me to my medical appointments. I also require steroid injections, as bub is likely to come any day now, and they want to ensure the lungs are strong enough.

We keep up the daily check-ins. At 37+1 weeks Dr Smalls makes the call that the baby needs to come out the following day.

It's a mad rush to organise Jeremy coming back from Brisbane, but we get it sorted.

I don't tell anyone aside from Dad, Jeremy, and a close friend what is happening. After the debacle of Xanthe's five day birth, I don't think I can handle it again.

Jeremy arrives home at 11pm on the 18th of June. At 6am the following morning we leave for Newcastle Private Hospital for a scheduled c-section.

As they prepare me for surgery, they send Jeremy to a waiting room telling him they will call him when it's time.

I am led down a corridor to have all my pre-op tests done. One of which includes weighing in.

I stare in dread at the scales. I haven't weighed in since seeing my old GP earlier in my pregnancy.

I was 145 kilograms then, will these scales even weigh me?

I know most scales have a weight limit of 150 kilograms. So I close my eyes and gingerly step on. Once again, I gingerly step on, as if it's going to magically alter the reading.

153 kilograms.

Fuck.

I barely register the rest of the pre-op routine as I sit in a fog.

153! How did I get to this?

Am I the fattest person ever to give birth?

I am led to the pre-op area.

As I am lying on the narrow bed waiting for the anaesthetist to come and attempt to put in my spinal block, I look down at my body. I really look at it for the first time in I can't remember how long.

Yes, I am pregnant. But I am also fat. Super unsustainably dangerously fat.

I am balanced precariously on this ridiculously narrow bed. I am too frightened to move a muscle less I fall to the floor. My breath is shallow just in case breathing too deeply causes me to move.

I am so scared that once they place the spinal block, and I can't feel my legs, I will lose my balance and topple to the floor, and they will need a crane or something to lift me back up.

I need to do something about this.

My brain replays every diet I have ever tried.

How long do I need to wait before doing something?

Should I rejoin the gym?

Does Weight Watchers still have local meetings?

Perhaps Tony Ferguson again to knock off some quick kilograms?

Should I try paleo?

As all these thoughts are racing through my mind, I feel a wave of frustrated exhaustion travel up my body.

I can't do this again. I am done with diets.

The anaesthetist arrives, takes one look at me, and

starts quoting statistics of spinal block success of someone of my size.

I honestly don't really hear most of what he says, because now I am almost at panic mode thinking about the upcoming delivery.

This is not Xanthe's birth. This is a new chance. You can do this.

Breathe. Just breathe.

Much to everyone's surprise the spinal block goes in first go, and Jeremy is finally allowed to join me as they wheel me into the theatre.

The music I asked for is playing, and I immediately begin to cry.

Each person introduces themselves. One midwife offers to play photographer, and takes the camera from Jeremy.

The general vibe in the room is so positive and uplifting. I feel like this can't possibly all be for me.

Suddenly my head splits open. Well, at least that's what it feels like. I swear someone has hit me in the head with a pick axe, and I immediately bring my hands to my head to remove the object I swear must be there.

I can hear the sound of screaming, and initially I don't register that the sound is coming from me.

"Suzanne, what's wrong?" a voice asks.

"My head. Make it stop. My head. Make it stop."

There are so many people in the room I barely register what is going on.

There is a flurry of movement around me. Someone brings in ice, lots of glorious ice packs, and places
them all around my head. The cooling sensation is
incredible.

The anaesthetist injects something into the cannula
on my wrist.

Blissfully the headache goes away.

What am I doing here? I want to go home.

I try to sit up, but my legs don't work. Frustrated, I
throw off the blanket.

"What are you doing?" asks Jeremy.

"I want to go home."

"WHAT?!?"

"I'm going home now."

"Ummmm, I think we are a bit committed now."

The realisation hits me. I am in the hospital about to
have my baby. I am instantly mortified.

"I'm sorry. I'm so sorry. I'm sorry. I'm sorry."

"Suzanne, it's totally ok. Are you ready for us to meet
this baby now? Can I begin?" Dr Smalls asks.

In that moment, I know this is going to be a whole
different experience from Xanthe.

"Yes."

I don't really feel a thing, not the pressure or the tug-
ging or the movement or any of the things I felt with
Xanthe. The music is exactly what I asked for. Everyone
is smiling, and reassuring me I am doing a great job.

I find it ironic that they say that, because I am hardly doing anything, just lying there. But I am so grateful for their comments, because I feel involved and part of the birth this time.

While I am revelling in this feeling. Dr Smalls says, "Dad get ready?"

"Ready for what?" I am confused.

"To cut the cord. It's time to meet bub."

"Already?"

Xanthe's birth had taken so long. Even the emergency cesarean part. I feel like Dr Smalls had only just opened me up.

The nurses lower the curtain so I can see. The midwife acting as photographer is wildly snapping pictures.

Dr Smalls lifts bub up slowly.

"It's a boy," he announces. Just like they do on TV shows.

"He's ok," I whisper in absolute relief and burst into tears.

Dr Smalls places him on my chest.

"Casimir," I say. I run my hand over his face, his skin is so soft and he is so very small, almost like a doll. I cradle him reverently and marvel that he is here and well. I can't wait for Xanthe to meet him.

The hospital stay following Casimir's birth is incredible. Aside from one midwife, the experience is absolutely beautiful. We stay for five nights.

On the morning of discharge as we are wheeling Casimir to the car, the nurse who is helping me along says, "It was lovely to have you. See you next time."

Which made me smile and laugh. While I am so grateful to have been so well looked after and cared for, I am done having babies.

Chapter Twelve

I am the heaviest I have ever been. But I cannot face another diet.

I am done.

I am sick of other people telling me what I can eat, how much, and when. I am sick of lists and plans and allowable and forbidden foods. I am sick of pills, powders and potions. I am sick of every new thing being 'The Thing'. I am sick of counting calories, points, macros, units. I am over it.

I walk calmly into the kitchen and I grab the biggest garbage bag I can find, and then I take it to my bedroom and I pick up every diet book, exercise book, every magazine, every guide, and I toss it in the bag.

As I try to move the bag, it rips under the weight of the books and I laugh at the irony of it.

I leave my room and search the garage for a big box and return, dumping all the books into it. I add my pedometers, my heart rate monitors, my fitbit and my garmin.

I add my stomach holding in undies, and my ab wave, the bosu and the weird things I bought that wrap around my arms that were supposed to get rid of my bingo wings.

The box is overflowing and still there are more things.

I clear a corner of the garage and begin to fill it with all the useless crap I have accumulated.

My back hurts. I'm tired. Yet still there is more to remove. Every last gimmick and gadget must go. I am never walking this path again.

At last it is all gone. My home is free of diet crap. My garage is a disaster zone. The thought of selling the stuff on gumtree briefly crosses my mind. There is literally thousands of dollars worth of stuff currently junking up my garage. But I can't face the effort of selling it. I just want it gone.

I collapse on the couch and burst into tears. I don't hold back. My shoulders shake, and I try not to make a sound lest I wake the baby. I don't know what I am going to do now.

No more dieting, now what?

I go to google and start typing in different search terms.

Weight loss mindset.

Lose weight without dieting.

Overcome emotional eating.

How to stop binge eating.

I come across a site by Kelly Reynolds. She talks about loving your body lean. It sounds preposterous, but I am intrigued.

Love your body, and it will become lean?

This is new.

Wow there are actually things I haven't come across before.
I thought I had seen it all.

I pour over her website. I read every article. I watch every video. I am totally engrossed. This sounds like exactly what I have been looking for. Something that's truly different to anything I've tried before.

Every other diet or program has been a variation of one I've done before. Whether it was counting calories, points, macros, or units. They have all talked about reducing food and increasing exercise.

This is different because it talks about mindset. The only other mindset stuff I have come across before was a brief mention in the 12WBT program, but this in depth.

There is a vague mention of a program, but no details. There are no prices listed on her site. I hate that. I like to know upfront what the costs are. The only option is to register for a body breakthrough call.

I spend a few days debating whether or not to book in the call.

What if I am not the right person, she says she is very selective about who she works with?

What if I am the right kind of person, and I really want it but I can't afford it?

After debating back and forth in my head for a few days, I book the call.

The call is scheduled for 2pm as I am hoping both my children will be napping and I can talk uninterrupted. I wake up early that morning feeling nervous and anxious.

It's one of those days where time seems to pass so slowly. I keep looking at the clock and hardly any time has passed at all. My mouth is dry just thinking about the call.

What if I say the wrong thing, and she doesn't want to work with me?

What if I am beyond help?

What if this doesn't work, and I am just going to be fat forever?

I am so worried I seriously consider cancelling the call. The debate rages in my head as I go between convincing myself I am beyond help to deciding that this is going to be 'The Thing.'

How many times have I thought that before. I am tired of my own bullshit.

By some miracle both children are napping at 2pm when the phone rings. I hold it in my hand watching it ring, debating not answering it.

Hurry up, and answer it before it wakes the kids.

"Hel-ahhh-Hi-this-is-Suzanne."

Great Robot voice, you've gotten this off to a great start.

"Hi Suzanne, great to connect with you. This is Kelly Reynolds, I am calling for your body breakthrough session, is now a good time?"

There is something about her tone that immediately relaxes me. It doesn't take long until we are talking like old friends. I feel relieved to have finally found someone who seems to 'get me'.

We talk for well over an hour.

We cover all the things I have tried before. This is a long list.

We discuss what worked, and what didn't. Deeper still, we cover what I liked, and what I didn't like, about each thing I have tried before. I really do begin to feel some clarity from just this discussion alone.

No wonder it's called a breakthrough session. Believe the hype.

"Do you want to know how we can do this together?" asks Kelly.

I am so very excited to hear the details. But equal parts feeling trepidation because I have already invested so much in my weight.

Is this going to be just another thing that doesn't work?

When Kelly mentions the price, I try to hide my gasp with a yawn.

"I've been up since 4am with the kids," I stutter to cover.

"What do you think?" Kelly asks.

"It sounds fabulous, but it really is out of my price range."

We discuss it for a few minutes. Kelly reminds me of all the reasons I really want this. While I agree with her, there is truly no way I can afford this. I am disappointed, but resigned.

Just when I think the conversation is over, and I am going to have to find something else, Kelly says there is another option. She will be running the program for a group, and I can do it that way rather than one to one, at a much reduced cost.

I feel a spark of hope. I ask how much it is, and it's still out of my price range. So she offers me a payment plan.

This is the biggest spend I have ever made on my health in one hit. It's even more expensive than the fat camp. I feel equal parts terrified and giddy as I read out my credit card number for her to set up the payment plan.

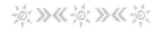

I start the program that very afternoon. I print out all of the resources and download all of the videos.

I am a bit confused.

Where are the lists of allowed and forbidden foods?

Where are all the prescribed exercise plans?

Why is there so much reference to journalling? I am a mum of two young kids, like I have time to journal.

What are these meditations? How is thinking about myself as a thin person going to work? It sounds totally bogus.

I begin to question my decision to sign up for this program. It feels foreign and overwhelming.

I try in vain to watch the videos, but my children never seem to sleep at the same time, so I find myself watching the same two minutes over and over again.

I begin to panic. I have invested so much into this, and I can't even get started.

That night when I put the kids to bed I sit down with my journal. I neatly write out the first journal prompt. Then I look at the blank page for what feels like hours. I notice the ink starting to smudge, and I realise that I am crying.

How has it come to this?

I've spent what feels like my whole life either doing exactly what I've been told, eat this, don't eat that, move that, stretch this, drink that. Now I am faced with looking at what is beyond all the food, and I feel lost?

I don't like where this is going. Sighing dejectedly, I head to the fridge. I will start again tomorrow.

The next day starts with me feeling more determined than ever before.

The first thing I do is upload all of the videos onto my ipod, that way I can listen to them while I walk. I load both kids into the double pram, and I head out the door.

It's a challenge to push the double pram. It's heavy. Xanthe keeps trying to leap out because she wants to walk. But apart from wriggling which makes the pram hard to steer, she is otherwise quiet.

I listen to the videos again and again. I love the sound of this mindset stuff.

Add more good things in, rather than cutting things out. I can do that.

Make sure that every meal has some form of protein, a good fat, and something fresh. I can do that.

Meditate twice per day. That's going to be hard. I can do once per day when the kids go to bed. I will start there.

Although the program doesn't say anything about weighing portion sizes, banishing junk foods, or anything like that. I do it anyway. I decide that this sounds too good to be true so I need to modify it.

I create my own diet. It feels liberating.

I follow my diet for three months, and I lose 24 kilograms. My weight loss has slowed down, and I am feeling frustrated. I am still 129 kilograms. What could I do to speed this up?

Later that day I catch up with a friend for morning tea. A lady called Kate introduces herself to us, and invites us to join a 12 week challenge at the local crossfit box. I smile and take the brochure, more to be polite than to really go. But the seed is planted.

I decide to join. But I don't tell anyone. I don't want anyone to see me fail, again.

Nervously, I turn up for the sign up class. I feel a bit like a neon michelin man. None of my workout gear fitted so I had to buy new items, and the only thing that came in my size is highlighter pink, and it sticks to every roll in a most unflattering way. Despite wanting to die of embarrassment and never leave my house again I force myself out the door.

The rules of this crossfit box are that every new participant must go to a three part beginners induction class. Because of the 12-week challenge, there are lots of new participants.

I quickly scan the room. I am the fattest person there, no surprise.

I am wondering if I can somehow sneak out unnoticed, wishing that my workout gear was camo instead of fluro-michelin man attire.

I wildly look around the room, wondering how I can cover my exit. I spot some protein powder looking things on the wall. Could I pretend that I had just come to buy one of those?

As I am formulating what I am going to say to make my grand escape I see a familiar face.

"Suzanne, I am so glad that you came," says Kate.

"Oh I am just here for the protein powder."

"Protein powder?" Kate raises her eyebrows.

"Yes." I say, pointing to the wall.

"Oh, honey, that's pre-workout." Kate smiles.

"Oh totally, I need that too." I say confidently, to cover my embarrassment. "I will just buy that and be on my way."

"So, you're not here to sign up for the challenge?"

"Oh no, just the preworkout."

"But what about your outfit? I love your workout gear. How about you just stay for this class, and then if you like, you can join in?" asks Kate.

I wish the floor would just swallow me up whole.

I stay for the class. I sign up for the 12 week challenge, and I leave feeling determined. This is going to be 'The Thing'.

I throw myself at crossfit with a single-minded focus. I ignore the pain, and the fact that my body hasn't done this for many years. I convince myself that 'muscle memory' will kick in soon, and that I just need to keep going.

My back starts to twinge, but I push through. *Just fucking do it*, becomes my mantra.

In the fourth week, I wake up one day and I am barely able to roll over out of bed. I feel like a turtle stuck lying on my back, and I imagine I must look like one, legs flailing around as I try without success to roll onto my side.

When rolling is unsuccessful, I kind of shimmy across the bed and try to swing my legs over the side. Instead I over balance and end up in a heap on the floor. *Fuck!*

I lay there in a daze for a few moments, before I manage to finally flip myself over and crawl to my bedside table. With more effort than I thought possible, I haul myself up to my feet. I stand there hunched over like an elderly woman, panting and trying to catch my breath.

"Waaaaaaaahhhhhh!"

Double fuck!

Somehow I struggle through the day with the kids, but I decide in that moment that crossfit isn't for me. I have been kidding myself. Maybe one day I could face it again. But trying to do something because I could do it in the past is crazy. I can see that now. Oh the wisdom of hindsight.

Over the following weeks my back doesn't improve. In fact it deteriorates rapidly. I have many more turtle moments, where I get stuck in bed. I also don't get a lot of sleep because when I lie down, I can't get comfortable.

I begin to withdraw from activities. I avoid catch ups with my friends. I avoid the library and the park with the kids. Everything hurts, and I just want to be alone.

I begin to eat more than ever before. Food doesn't ask me questions, food doesn't cry or complain or demand. Food is just there, and for a moment, a very brief moment, it makes me feel better.

One night when the kids are in bed I am sitting on the couch watching DVDs and slamming my way through a family block of chocolate, when I reach for a piece and feel just the crinkle of the wrapper.

I look down and realise that I am staring at an empty wrapper.

Mother fucker! I didn't get to enjoy the last piece.

I haul myself off the couch and storm into the kitchen throwing open the pantry.

No chocolate.

I check all the draws and wander around the house searching all my usual hiding places.

Still no chocolate.

Fuck.

I look at the clock. It's 9pm. Woolies would still be open.

I would have to wake the kids.

Shit. Shit. Shit.

I am standing there, debating what to do.

What the hell are you doing to yourself?

An inner argument ensues.

I didn't get to enjoy the last piece. My inner 3 year old rages.

Are you serious? There's my inner adult.

Calm down, let's think about this rationally. My inner peacekeeper chimes in.

While this is all going on, and I am questioning my own sanity, I have a flash of realisation.

I didn't get to enjoy the last piece. What about the other like fifty pieces of the block?

I am floored.

THE BEGINNING IS SH*T

What about the other fifty pieces? Why did only the last piece count?

This had never occured to me before.

In all the years, and all the diets, and all the things I had tried and followed, no one had ever asked me such a simple question.

I go to bed still mulling this over.

Chapter Thirteen

My weight is all over the show. I have 'good' food weeks and 'bad' food weeks.

Throughout it all my back is absolutely killing me. I have many more 'turtle' moments.

I'm SO tired but I can't sleep. Between my back and Casimir's constant wailing, I don't know how I make it through each day.

Casimir is six months old and doesn't like to lie down. He has to be held upright constantly. It's the only thing that settles him. For someone with a bad back this is torture.

I take Casimir to my GP, then a paediatrician, and he is finally diagnosed with silent reflux.

Children's Gaviscon is liquid gold!

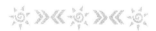

I'm sitting on the couch, the kids are on the floor, the Wiggles are on TV, and the next minute Casimir has pulled himself up on the lounge, he's almost one.

Oh no, buddy, Mummy's not ready for this…

Before I can even finish my thought Casimir topples to the ground and he's howling.

As he falls, I rush to scoop him up and my back spasms. I collapse alongside him and start crying too.

Xanthe, looking from me to Casimir and back to me, starts wailing too.

As I lie on the ground surrounded by tears and snot, I wonder.

How am I going to do this?

I can barely keep up with Xanthe, and now Casimir is about to start walking.

These thoughts continue to plague me, even keeping me up at night.

I can't go on like this so I go to see my GP about my back pain.

First she sends me for a plain X-ray, next a CT scan, and finally she orders an MRI.

I call to book my MRI appointment, deciding brutal honesty is the best approach.

"Not only am I highly claustrophobic, but I also seriously doubt my ability to fit into the MRI machine. Can you please book me into a bigger machine? I don't mind travelling," I tell the receptionist.

"Oh don't worry, dear, you'll be fine," she reassures me.

"Seriously, I weigh around 150 kilograms. Can you please book me into a bigger machine?" I plead.

"You'll be fine, I will book you into our Maitland clinic," she says.

Bloody Maitland again. This suburb has it in for me.

On the day of the appointment I front up to the clinic with some trepidation.

When my name is called I can see the technician sizing me up mentally.

"Ummmmmmm." she begins hesitantly.

"I'm not sure that our facility is the best place for you. We have a larger machine in Newcastle," she says delicately.

"Great, when can I book in?" I say in relief.

"Oh, don't worry!" comes a booming voice from across the room. "We can make her fit. I'm good at tetris," says a jovial young man.

Run! My inner voice screams.

I ignore my better judgement and follow the pair into the room.

They have to rearrange my body like a bloody contortionist as they grab parts of my flab and shove, using small pillows to wedge me in.

It takes what feels like eternity and four technicians to jam me into the MRI machine.

I am mortified and in pain as they place the earphones over my ears.

"Remember, I'm claustrophobic," I remind them.

"Don't worry your head doesn't go in," someone tells me as they all file out of the room. "Be sure to keep still, or we will have to rebook you into the machine at Newcastle."

I wish the bloody receptionist had just booked me in there to begin with like I had asked.

As my body slowly rolls into the machine, I'm silently panicking and debating pressing the button to bail. I'm crying, but silent tears to keep as still as possible. It's taken them over 20 minutes to jam me into this machine. I don't want to go through this all over again.

As my chin starts to go in and I can no longer see the ceiling I'm silently cursing them for lying about my head not going in, but then it stops at my nose.

We have a very different definition of a covered head.

The next day I visit my GP again. I'm referred to a neurosurgeon. I make the appointment, and thankfully I'm able to attend while the kids are at daycare.

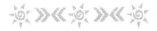

It's hot. It is so ridiculously hot in this waiting room, and I am watching the clock, and praying that this neurosurgeon isn't running too far behind.

I am in so much pain. My back is killing me, and I need to get out of here in 30 minutes, or I won't be able to pick up my kids from daycare on time.

Why are doctors so notoriously late when it feels like you are only ever in their rooms for a moment?

"Suzanne Culberg?"

I hear my name being called, and I struggle to pull myself up from the low couch.

"I've reviewed your scans," he begins, "and I think the best course of action is spinal fusion surgery...."

He continues on discussing the procedures. It would be a two-part surgery. I would need at least six weeks of support, and I'm not really hearing him as my mind is going a hundred miles an hour.

What about my kids? Who is going to look after them while I recover?

What if it doesn't work?

What if I die on the table?

"….50% chance you won't need the surgery….." he continues.

"Wait? What?" I interrupt him.

"If you weren't so overweight then there is a 50% chance you wouldn't need the surgery," he repeats.

This has caught my attention.

He continues to discuss the ins and outs of the procedure, but my mind keeps mulling over the weight loss side of it.

I head out of the appointment, pick the kids up from daycare and head straight to the supermarket. I stock up on healthy foods.

Once the kids are asleep I empty out the fridge, freezer and pantry.

I dig out my old recipe books, grab a pad and paper, and draw up a menu plan for dinners. This is it. It's time. I'm finally ready.

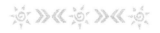

None of my clothes fit.

I literally only have a handful of items of clothing.

Despite my new resolve and efforts, I haven't lost any weight yet. I'm feeling a bit despondent to be making all these changes and not seeing any results yet.

In the past I refused to buy new clothes until I've lost weight. OR I buy new clothes in smaller sizes and hang them in strategic places to 'motivate' myself.

Except if I am truly honest, it has never motivated me.

Every time I look at a beautiful outfit that doesn't fit I am reminded of how fat I currently am, and that usually sends me off in a shame spiral that ends with me pigging out.

Not this time. I resolve to buy clothes that actually fit.

I drop the kids off at daycare early in the morning and head into Newcastle.

By lunch time, I'm frustrated, close to tears and questioning my choices.

Nothing fits me anywhere.

Not even the XL in the plus sized shops.

You know you're big when even fat fashions no longer caters to you.

Eventually I end up in Myers.

I am equal parts excited to see that their clothes fit and horrified by the price tag.

All the old thoughts of waiting till I've lost weight, or buying clothes in the next size down start to fill my head.

I don't want to waste money.

I will lose weight soon. I don't need that much.

I listen to these voices, and decide FUCK IT and buy the clothes anyway.

I spend well over a thousand dollars, and come home with pants that don't cut into me, bras that I don't want to rip off as soon as I walk in the door and a totally new lease on life.

Chapter Fourteen

I decide to document the process.

Baseline stats, I'm going to need weight, measurements and photographs. I decide to weigh in weekly, and then re-do measurements and photos monthly.

With trepidation I walk into my bathroom and dust off my scales. I stand on it and see the numbers flash to 150kg.

I sigh. Here I am again.

I knew it was going to be bad, but I don't freak out like I would have in the past. I retrieve a journal and write down the date, my weight, and create columns for my measurements.

I feel a sense of calm as I go through this familiar starting stats routine.

I retrieve a measuring tape, and measure my neck, chest, upper arm, and write each number in the corresponding column.

When I get to my belly the measuring tape won't go all the way round.

Fuck.

The measuring tape maxes out at 150cm and there is a lot more belly than there is tape.

I decide to draw on my belly with a pen, mark where the tape gets to, and then measure the gap.

15cm.

That means I am 165cm around my waist.

I am literally as round as I am tall.

This sounds like the start of a bad country music tune.

Maybe I will one day be famous for writing a ditty about my size.

Despondently, I finish off my measurements: hips, thighs, calves.

In the past I've done my measurements and headed straight to the fridge.

This time I just sit there.

What now?

I reflect on my time with Kelly, all I had learnt about mindset, and how I told myself at the time I wasn't dieting, how I had inadvertently turned it into a diet.

As the saying goes 'old habits die hard.'

I can't face another diet.

I mean it this time.

I reflect on ALL the things I've tried in the past.

I realise I need to do something different.

I recall a quote "If you want something you've never had. You must be willing to do something you've never done."

Where to start?

Hunger.

How is this different?

Well in the past I've always started with food. What I was eating. This time I was starting with hunger.

I had learnt a lot about hunger in the past, from diets, from books, from programs. But I had never truly applied any of it.

Honestly, hunger scared me. I was scared that if I allowed myself to get hungry I would never stop eating.

I felt the constant need to eat 'in case' I got hungry. So I had no real frame of reference for what hunger truly felt like.

I decided that I would give my hunger a scale.

Where -10 was starving, so hungry that I would eat kale. To me, kale tasted like I would rather be fat!

And +10 was stuffed, like post-Christmas lunch, and you-have-to-undo-the-button-on-your-pants-and-roll-yourself-away-from-the-table-stuffed.

Before I ate anything, I would check in with myself and where I was on the hunger scale.

Immediately after eating anything I would check in again, and where I was on the hunger scale.

At first this was really challenging.

All my fears about being hungry came up.

I keep having flashbacks to my past shake diets, and my body trim days, and convincing myself that this was never going to work.

But I kept reminding myself this was NOT a diet. I was not changing WHAT I ate, all I was doing was checking in with myself where I was on my hunger scale and committing to not eating until I felt hungry, so I had to be in the negatives on the scale.

I felt a freedom I had never known before, because nothing was restricted. I could truly eat whatever I wanted, whenever I wanted it, provided I was actually hungry.

I eat a lot, and I mean A LOT of cookie dough.

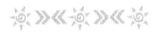

After four weeks of committing to eating only when I'm hungry, I weigh in at five kilos heavier than when I started.

I am sitting on the couch, feeling defeated and watching the kids play on the floor, and I feel an unfamiliar feeling, in the pit of my stomach.

It feels like a craving.

It can't be that. You haven't had any cravings since you gave up dieting. What's there to crave anyway? You're practically living on cookie dough.

I sit with the feeling for a bit longer, trying to work out what it could possibly be.

No, it's most definitely a craving.

A craving for what? You have eaten everything and then some over the last month.

I realise that I feel like broccoli.

Say what now?! You crave broccoli. Who are you, and what have you done with the real Suzanne?

I drag my astonished self from the couch, round up the kids and head to the supermarket. It's vegetable time.

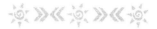

It feels really rather liberating to learn to get in touch with my hunger signals.

But the commitment to eat only when hungry isn't as easy as I had first thought.

Learning the difference between hungry and hangry is a process.

I realise in the past what I thought was hungry, was actually hangry, and once I reach a certain point I am 'too far gone' so to speak, and so of course I overeat.

It seems kind of logical when I look at it through this lens, rather than with a dieting focus.

Some days I eat constantly, and other days hardly anything at all.

This freaks me out in the beginning.

By not eating am I going to kill my metabolism?

I've always been told I need to fuel the fire.

By eating constantly am I not giving my body a break?

Is this going to work?

My anxiety levels are high!

It takes about six months for me to truly learn what hunger feels like, how it starts as a little niggle under my rib, and then from there becomes a pulse in my chest.

If I eat at this point, I really don't need much food.

However, if I let it progress, it becomes a growl in my stomach, then a light headed feeling, and then my hands start to shake and I become snappy. By then I am too far gone — hello hangry!

It's incredible how freeing this process is.

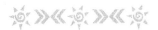

Now at the six month point so much has changed. I no longer weigh in weekly. I found the weekly weigh-in process disheartening because, on average, I would only lose weight one week per month.

In a typical month I would stay the same weight for two weeks, gain one week thanks to 'that time of the month' and then lose four kilos in the next week.

So overall my average monthly weight loss was three kilograms, but instead it looked like, week one same, week two same, week three gain one kilogram, week four lose four kilograms.

As a result I change my process to monthly weigh-ins, photographs, and measurements. It seems easier to do this all together once per month.

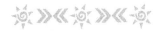

I feel it's time to try something new so I review some of my mindset material, and I choose to 'add things in.'

I decide that I can still eat whatever I want, but I need to eat some 'good' things at each meal.

I don't like how I have delineated food into 'good' and 'bad.' I've thought about food this way for as long as I can remember, but it doesn't sit well with me any longer.

Because to me, if I eat 'bad' food, then I am a 'bad' person. I no longer like this connotation.

Instead of 'good' food, I choose to say 'nourishing' food. This feels like a small but important shift in my thinking.

Using this 'adding' principle, I can still eat whatever I want as long as I've eaten something nourishing first.

So if I crave chocolate, I first have some fruit and yogurt, or some dip and carrot sticks, and then if I still want the chocolate I have it.

At first I am still eating most of a block of chocolate each day. But it's not long before this reduces significantly.

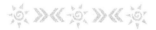

While eating only when hungry and adding things in is going surprisingly well, I can't help feeling like I am wasting a lot of food.

As someone who was brought up to 'finish everything on your plate as there are starving children in Africa' it is feeling very wasteful to stop eating as soon as I feel satisfied. Because now that I am being honest with myself, this is taking an alarmingly small amount of food.

There are times when I am really enjoying something, the taste, the smell, the texture, that I just don't want to stop.

When I put the food down on my plate and walk away, it's almost like it's calling me.

Or if I am out at a restaurant, and I see it sitting there on the plate, I can't stop thinking *I've paid good money for this, eat up!*

Who came up with the idea of 'good money' anyway? What would it be like to pay 'bad money' for something? I will shelve that thought for another day.

There are many times that I struggle to stop eating.

I try many strategies. I portion the food out and put some away in the fridge or the pantry.

Only to find myself there thirty minutes later eating it all.

I order smaller serves or buy smaller amounts. But if I am honest, often even the smaller serves are too much for me.

There has to be something else I can do.

Day care is having a pie drive. I look at this list of options and say to myself -

Order nothing, just make a donation, that is the smart thing to do.

As I scan the list I see vanilla slice as an option.

Vanilla slice is my kryptonite. I want it, and I want it now.

I order one, telling myself that I am supporting the day care.

The following week the vanilla slice arrives and it is humongous. It's more like a vanilla cake than a slice.

I take my first bite, and it is sensational. Like a party in my mouth. Hands down THE best vanilla slice I have ever eaten. However after merely a few bites I realise I feel satisfied.

Well that was a let down.

I dutifully put the vanilla slice back in the fridge and go about my business.

Well, I try to go about my business. I swear I can hear it calling me. Every few minutes I find myself with the door open staring longingly into the fridge.

I swear it's like a siren calling me to my doom.

Finally I take it out of the fridge, telling myself *Just one more bite won't hurt.*

In that moment I feel like I'm at a precipice. Will I give into my old ways and go down this road knowing that one bite will become two, will become the whole thing, washed down with ice cream and whatever else I can find, all the while telling myself *I'll start again tomorrow?*

Or will I ride this out?

For some reason an old saying comes to mind, "Old ways won't open new doors."

In that moment I open the pantry, grab the barbeque sauce and dump it all over the top of the vanilla slice.

There. I won't eat it now.

As I clean up the mess, scraping the ruined vanilla slice into the bin and thinking -

What a waste.

I'm also contemplating that, had I eaten it, it would have ended up on my literal waist.

Waste or waist? Either way it's wasted.

I like the sound of this mantra, waste or waist — you decide? I commit to using this going forward.

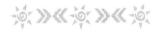

At the twelve month mark, I know it's time to begin to do something more than just walking. I've lost thirty kilograms, but that still has me weighing in at 120 kilograms.

It's disheartening that no one has really noticed my weight loss. Or if they have, they haven't commented.

Although I feel disappointed that I don't really look that different on the outside. I do feel appreciative that I haven't had to give up any of my favourite foods or bust my ass at the gym.

Reintroducing exercise is something I'm reluctant to do.

I know the health benefits. I also know the pain and humiliation of my past.

Walking back into the gym is a mixed bag of emotions. Part of me is embarrassed that I have let myself get to this size, and part of me feels at home.

It's the smell, as weird as it sounds. I love the smell of the gym, that mix of sweat and metal and deodorant. It makes me feel committed just smelling it!

You are one gross fucked up individual Suze!

The first class I attend is body balance.

I will ease into it with one of my old favourites.

Back in the day I used to do Body Balance as a recovery class on the back of Pump or Spin.

I start the class with great zeal, only to realise after the warm up that I'm in trouble.

I can't even make it through the warm up, what the fuck have I become?

I struggle my way through the class.

There are so many movements I can't do either due to my sheer size or my back.

I can't even lie on the floor.

Why did I think this was a good idea?

At the end of the class I'm trying my best to hide my tears and make my way out as fast as I can. When I hear, "Hey is that you, Suze?"

Fuck!

I look up to see a mum from daycare whose name I can't recall. I pretend to sneeze to cover my tears and as she makes her way over to me I say, "Oh allergies."

I don't register the conversation. I never have been one for small talk. But at the end she is smiling at me saying

"See you back here next week?"

"Sure," I lie. And head to my car as fast as my sore, tired body will carry me.

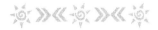

Realising I am too unfit for even the most basic of group fitness classes throws a total spanner in the works.

What do I do now?

I start walking laps of the pool. Everything else hurts too much.

After a few months of this, I brave another group fitness class. This time I try water aerobics.

I am both the youngest and fattest in the pool.

I am also the slowest.

Wow these oldies are showing me how it's done!

I start with one class a week, then two.

Eventually, I brave a yoga class again.

After 11 months back at the gym I'm finally able to lie flat on my back.

I cry. This time happy tears. It feels so good.

As my fitness continues to improve, I cautiously attempt body pump. Then circuit. Then body attack.

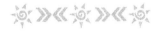

I've been plodding along for nearly two years now. Jeremy is still working away in Sydney. I am working from home part time as a personal assistant while the kids are at day-care three days per week.

I'm feeling much more confident in my process as I've dropped just over 50 kilograms.

Many people are asking me for advice and wanting to know what it is that I'm doing. I start to share more openly on facebook about my journey.

I share photos, quotes, and my thoughts about what it is that I am learning. I also decide to write a weekly newsletter.

The first week I have four subscribers. Two of them are my mum and sister, but nevertheless I'm both excited and nervous to share.

Each week the number of people following me on facebook and joining my newsletter grows, and I love having the external accountability to keep taking action.

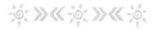

Having lost a significant amount of weight twice before this attempt, I know that chances are I'm going to need a tummy tuck at the end of this process.

Back when I lost the 43kg and then again when I lost the 60kg, excess skin was an issue. It's being compounded this time by the fact that I've now also had two children.

I know a surgery of this nature is going to cost a pretty penny and although we're comfortable, we are not the kind of folks who have a lazy ten grand just lying around.

I know if I want this procedure I'm going to have to be a bit creative.

"Start a go fund me page," my sister insists.

"Ummmmm that's the kind of thing people do when a house burns down or if someone is sick," I reply.

"You will sure as hell be sick after a tummy tuck," she jokes.

"Not the same thing," I say and change the subject so we chat about something else.

But my brain is still churning.

How am I going to afford this?

The following day I'm at the supermarket, and I'm totally hanging out for a chocolate.

It's like magic, one minute I'm thinking about chocolate and the next I have a family block in my trolley.

As I reluctantly put the block back on the shelf I notice the price, five dollars, and I tell myself I've just saved $5. I wonder how much this lifestyle change is saving me.

In that moment a thought occurs to me. What about if every time I reach for chocolate, or coke, or some other form of junk food, where in the past I would have bought it, I put that money aside towards my tummy tuck?

This sounds like a great idea. But a week later I notice I haven't actually made any progress towards starting.

I decide to make a new account with a separate bank to my usual institution. That way I won't be tempted to either spend the money or fob it off like I have for the last week.

I create a new bank account. I save the details into my app, and from that day, whenever I feel tempted to buy any junk food, I look at how much it costs, I immediately open my banking app and transfer the funds across to my other account.

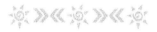

Once I've dropped 58 kilograms, my personal assistant contract is terminated. I'm gutted. I put my heart and soul into that role, and now I have nothing.

My first thought is to go back to my call centre job. But with Jeremy still in Sydney, getting two kids into daycare and driving over an hour to the call centre is not appealing.

I'm literally sitting on the floor crying about losing my job when Kelly, the mindset coach, emails me.

"Hey Suze, I've been following your facebook page. Damn girl you look fabulous! Have you thought about coaching? I would love for you to work for us. You'd just need to complete a coach certification. It just so happens we have one coming up; let me know if you'd like some deets."

Talk about divine timing.

Chapter Fifteen

The coach certification is a ten month program with both online and in-person trainings.

While I enjoy the in-person training it means that I don't get to see Jeremy at all those weekends. We are literally like ships passing in the night, as he comes home to take the children, and I travel to Sydney for training.

We decide that he and the kids should join me for one of the weekend workshops. He will take care of the kids during the day, going to the park or the aquarium, and then we will catch up together as a family in the evening.

We book into a two bedroom apartment in Darling Harbour. The kids and I catch the train into the city and meet up with Jeremy after work. After a quick stop in at Coles supermarket, we make our way to the hotel to check in.

The kids run off exploring as Jeremy and I unpack our groceries in the kitchen. Next minute Casimir comes racing into the kitchen.

"Mummy there's a baaaaaaad man in my room," he says unsteadily.

We run into his room.

There, we are greeted with a large picture of Luna Park at night.

We both collapse into giggles.

I look over at Jeremy who is still holding a carton of milk.

"What were you planning to do, bludgeon the bad man with a milk carton?" I ask, laughing hysterically.

He looks over at me. "What were you going to do, make him a sandwich?"

I look down to see I'm still holding a loaf of bread.

We collapse into giggles, relieved that there is no intruder to deal with.

Later that night, once the kids are finally asleep, I decide to have a bath. There is an enormous bath tub and bubble bath. I feel like I'm in seventh heaven.

I read until long after the bath has gone cold, and when I come out of the bathroom all the lights are off.

Realising that Jeremy must have gone to sleep, I attempt to sneak quietly across the apartment less I wake him or the kids.

Using the torch function on my phone I pick my way across the room, wondering how there can be so much stuff all over the floor in the short time we've been here.

Kids are like mini tornadoes, I think as I dodge yet another toy.

As silently as possible I ease open the bedroom door, enter quietly, and close it softly behind me. As I look up to step away from the door, the phone light catches a figure lurking. I drop the towel and scream loudly.

It takes a moment to register that the figure has also dropped a towel.

Oh my goodness this is me.

I've lost so much weight that I don't recognise myself. Meanwhile Jeremy has jumped up in bed and is slurring disorientedly, "Who....Whaaaaat....you ok?"

"All good, go back to sleep," I tell him.

The next morning he teases me about this moment relentlessly. I realise I won't live this down anytime soon.

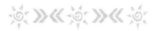

I've now lost 70 kilograms, and I get mixed reactions from my friends and family.

Some are genuinely happy for me and supportive.

Others start to ply me with treats while saying things like "just one won't hurt."

Then there are the people who tell me they're concerned about my well-being and say things such as, "You're not going to lose anymore are you? You're starting to look gaunt."

Some people stop inviting me to events, and I hear comments like "I didn't think you'd be interested because of your diet."

I'm not on a diet. My frustration is palpable.

Would it be cocky to invite them to follow me on face-book so they see what it actually is that I'm doing?

At a time where I thought I would feel amazing I feel so alone.

I find more and more that, now I'm no longer the 'fat friend,' people don't relate to me anymore.

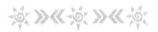

Spice and Lime is the most amazing Thai restaurant in Singleton. One night I'm meeting my good friends Abby and John there for dinner.

We haven't seen each other in a few years, so I'm excited to catch up. I arrive at the restaurant early and grab the table.

I look up and see John at the door.

I wave madly at him. No response.

I yell at him across the room, and it's like he doesn't even hear me.

I rush over to him, say "Hi" and go in for the hug, and he jumps back yelling "I'm married!"

Next thing Abby comes up behind him, laughing hysterically, saying, "Hi Suzanne."

John's face goes from red, to purple, to white as he stutters, "I honestly didn't recognise you, Suze. You look like a totally different person."

Chapter Sixteen

My ultimate goal on every weight loss attempt has been a flat stomach. Unfortunately releasing 75 kilograms has left me with a large amount of loose skin around my waist.

A number of well meaning people tell me "you don't need surgery, you just need to do some sit ups," and then I lift up my shirt and watch their eyes bulge.

I am hesitant to have the procedure because it's a significant expense and I feel extravagant spending that much money on myself. Not to mention the risks involved, what if something goes wrong? The procedure is elective. I don't really need it.

I book an initial appointment with a surgeon to discuss my options, and he quotes me five thousand dollars.

I check the balance of my second bank account where I have been squirreling away my funds each time I'm tempted to buy junk food, and I'm pleasantly surprised to discover I have saved just over three thousand dollars. This makes it imminently affordable, and we set a date for the procedure.

※ 》《 ※ 》《 ※

The day of the surgery arrives. We drop the kids off to daycare, and Jeremy drives me into the hospital in the city.

The early morning traffic is heavy, and so he's busy concentrating on the road while I'm freaking out and changing my mind what feels like a billion times, although deep down inside I want this more than anything.

My phone rings. It's my mum.

"Hey Suze, how are you going?" she asks.

"Well, Mum, I'm freaking out and changing my mind repeatedly."

We chat back and forth for a few minutes and just as she hangs up the phone she says "Love you," and I immediately burst into tears.

"Turn the car around." I say to Jeremy.

"Wait! What? Why?" he stammers, eyes glued to the road.

"I'm going to die." I wail adamantly.

"Huh?" he asks, confused and distracted.

"Well, all my life Mum has never said she loved me. I asked her about it once, and she said whenever she told anyone she loved them, they died and so she never says 'love you'."

"So what?" he asks.

"Soooooooooooooooooooo!" I shriek. "She just told me on the phone she loves me so that means I'm going to die! So let's go home now!"

This all makes perfect sense to me. I don't know why he's taking so long to catch on, and I'm really starting to panic now, and am debating grabbing the steering wheel to show him that I'm serious when he says, "The old you will die and the new you will be reborn."

Instantly my tears dry up, and I think this is the most profound thing my husband has ever said to me.

"Keep driving," I murmur.

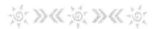

Many hours later as they wheel me onto the ward post surgery, I'm groggy and disoriented when a kind nurse says, "Oh, Mrs Culberg, here you are. We've been waiting for you. I just spoke to your husband. He rang to check on you. He will be happy to know you're here. You've been in recovery for seven hours."

Seven hours? Holy shit! Am I ok?

I drift in and out of sleep. I can't see anything clearly. I vaguely remember asking for my glasses. I don't know what time it is. Hell, I don't know what day it is.

Eventually my brain starts to clear. I reach for my phone and see it's 10pm. I'm finally coherent enough to have a conversation with the nurse. It turns out they've lost my glasses, but she's confident they will find them. More importantly she explains the pain button to me. I press that thing like a kid playing whack-a-mole.

The next morning it's time for me to get out of bed. The nurse arrives, removes my cannula, explains to me to be mindful of the drains, and talks me through the process of getting up.

I've had two C-sections, how bad can it be?

I start to move and…

Holy Fucking Hell this is absolute agony! I feel like I'm literally being sawn in half! Please for the love of all things make it stop!

"Can't," I manage to pant out.

"I'm not leaving this room till you get out of bed, Mrs Culberg," she says in a kind tone.

Well, you're going to be here a long fucking time!

Eventually I made it out of bed.

But that was without a doubt THE most fucking painful experience of my life.

I assumed the recovery from my tummy tuck would be similar to my C-sections, improving significantly each day.

I was wrong.

I return home after five nights in hospital, and the first night at home is pure hell.

I cannot lie down in my bed; it's too low and too flat.

Unlike the hospital, I can't change the height or the recline.

I can't even cry because that hurts.

I'm in a hell of my own making. No one understands, or rarely cares. At least that is how it seems.

"You chose this. It's what you wanted," my dad reminds me unhelpfully.

I'm exhausted and emotional and probably beyond reason. I'm eight days post surgery, I haven't really slept since I left the hospital and the panadol I'm taking is doing nothing for the pain.

It's moments like these where I wish I weren't allergic to fucking everything.

Nothing is working to ease my pain, so out of pure desperation, I put on a meditation.

I don't know why it has taken me this long to think of it as I have been an avid meditator for the past three years.

For a few blissful moments I feel absolutely nothing…and finally I drift off to sleep.

※ 》《 ※ 》《 ※

The recovery from the tummy tuck is much longer and harder than I anticipated.

All in all they had removed 3.3 kilograms of excess skin, taking my total weight loss to 78 kilograms.

Thankfully there are no complications or infections, and once the pain settles down, I begin to feel human again.

After two weeks my drains are removed.

At the three week mark all my dressings come off.

The scar is jagged and long. I had heard that it would be 'hip to hip' but I thought that meant just across my front.

Instead it goes over the back of each hip, so that literally only a palms-width of skin at the back is uncut.

"I look like a magician tried to saw me in half and botched the job," I say to Jeremy.

"I'm so glad your sense of humour is returning," he replies.

By six weeks, I'm allowed to ditch the compression garments and I can finally stand upright.

I never thought I'd see the day when shaving under my arms made me feel human again, but there you have it.

At my final post-op appointment the bandages are finally all removed and I can see my stomach in the mirror.

The apron of hanging skin is finally gone, and I have the flat stomach that I had always dreamed of.

Epilogue

It's been just over three years since my tummy tuck.

I'm finishing the first draft of this book at a beautiful resort on the Sunshine Coast. Ironically, it's actually just down the road from where I went to fat camp all those years ago.

Jeremy has been through two more redundancies, and we have undertaken two more interstate moves. Let me tell you, they are a lot more rocky with children added to the mix.

Xanthe is nearly eight, and it will be Casimir's birthday next week. He will turn six.

Reliving my life story through creating this book has been an epic roller coaster of emotions. I have laughed, cried, gone to the fridge, headed out for a walk and nearly quit, repeatedly. But here we are at the end.

I still use all the mindset tools I mentioned in this book, and many more I continue to learn along the way.

I still have times where I don't make the best food decisions, and find myself at the fridge or pantry. But instead of beating myself up, I use these moments to show myself true compassion, and look for where I need to lean in and look after myself even more.

In sharing my story the biggest thing that has stood out for me was that with every weight loss attempt I started I was always convinced it was going to be 'The Thing.'

What I can now recognise is that signing up for any program with the energy of 'this is going to be The Thing that solves my problem' is where the issue lies.

It has taken trying to fix myself repeatedly to realise that fixing myself wasn't that answer because I was never broken.

What IS broken is societal conditioning that our self worth is tied to our clothing size, and that food has to be earned, and exercise is seen as a punishment. My thoughts about this may well be the topic of my next book.

If I had to sum what I have learned throughout this whole journey into five statements they would be…

1. You are allowed to be both a masterpiece and a work in progress at the same time.
2. What you do today matters. Who you are today is the result of the decisions you made a year ago. Who you are a year from now is the result of the decisions you make today.
3. You can't hate yourself happy, or punish yourself skinny. You can't do all the things you loathe and expect to live a life you love. Food and exercise are both sources of nourishment, not things to be earned or controlled.

4. There is no before, there is no after, there is only ever now.
5. You must show up for yourself. When you make showing up for yourself a non-negotiable priority, that's when the game changes.

If you're not ready to say goodbye, there is more awaiting you here:

www.suzanneculberg.com/bonus

If you see yourself in my story and would like to explore working together further, I invite you to check out my coaching offerings on my website:

www.suzanneculberg.com

My clients affectionately call me the velvet hammer, equal parts caring and cattle prod.

If you have enjoyed this book, please don't keep it a secret, share it with a friend.

Thank you for taking the time to read this story. It has been an honour to share my experiences, both the highs and lows with you. My hope is that you feel renewed hope for your own journey, and wherever you are right now, remember while the beginning is shit, the rest is still unfolding.

About the Author

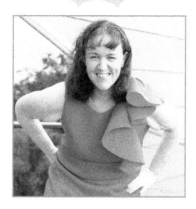

SUZANNE CULBERG is an international mindset coach for women seeking weight loss based in Sydney, Australia. She believes that women often gain too much weight themselves because they give too much help to others. They over-eat because they over-give. Suzanne's passion for helping women is fueled by her own weight loss journey, going from 150kg to maintaining the healthy 72kg she is now.

Suzanne lives with her husband Jeremy and her two young children who keep her both busy and entertained. When she's not coaching her clients, running her programs, sharing her latest bit of wisdom on Facebook Live, podcasting or writing her popular newsletter, she can be found reading, enjoying Diamond Dotz, or burlesque dancing. She is also a big fan of yoga.

Learn more about Suzanne at **www.suzanneculberg.com** or find her on YouTube at **https://suzanneculberg.com/youtube.**

CPSIA information can be obtained
at www.ICGtesting.com
Printed in the USA
BVHW081438230921
617401BV00001B/72

9 780645 274905